ST
FO
AN
CA   S

STUDY SKILLS FOR HEALTH AND SOCIAL CARE STUDENTS

JULIETTE OKO
JAMES REID

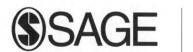
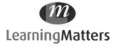

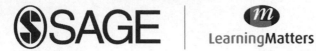
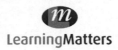

Learning Matters
An imprint of SAGE Publications Ltd
1 Oliver's Yard
55 City Road
London EC1Y 1SP

SAGE Publications Inc.
2455 Teller Road
Thousand Oaks, California 91320

SAGE Publications India Pvt Ltd
B 1/I 1 Mohan Cooperative Industrial Area
Mathura Road
New Delhi 110 044

SAGE Publications Asia-Pacific Pte Ltd
3 Church Street
#10-04 Samsung Hub
Singapore 049483

Editor: Luke Block
Development editor: Lauren Simpson
Production controller: Chris Marke
Project management: Swales & Willis Ltd,
Exeter, Devon
Marketing manager: Tamara Navaratnam
Cover design: Wendy Scott
Typeset by: Swales & Willis Ltd, Exeter, Devon
Printed by: MPG Books Group, Bodmin,
Cornwall

Library of Congress Control Number:
2012936249

British Library Cataloguing in Publication Data

A catalogue record for this book is available
from the British Library

ISBN 978 0 85725 874 8
ISBN 978 0 85725 805 2 (pbk)

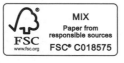

Contents

About the authors   vi

Introduction   1

1 Learning to learn   5

2 Verbal and non-verbal communication skills   18

3 Information literacy, thinking, reading and writing   33

4 Developing presentation skills   56

5 Practice learning and ethical practice   69

6 Understanding and using reflection   83

Conclusion   97

Glossary   99

References   105

Index   108

About the authors

Juliette Oko is a Senior Lecturer and Associate Teaching Fellow at Teesside University. She teaches on the undergraduate programme in social work and is also the admissions tutor for the course. Her interests include teaching and learning and reflective practice. Prior to entering academia, she worked as a qualified social worker in the field of adults and mental health and children and families social work. She is also the author of the successful textbook, *Understanding and Using Theory in Social Work*, published by Learning Matters.

James Reid is a Senior Lecturer in Childhood Studies in the School of Education and Professional Development at the University of Huddersfield. He is a registered social worker and a Fellow of the Higher Education Academy in the UK. James has contributed to several textbooks on health and social care and social work, most recently on international perspectives of children and the law.

INTRODUCTION

This book is aimed at readers who are interested in the subject of health and social care or early years and childhood studies and are thinking of going to university or college to study this subject or who may be beginning their studies in, say, a foundation degree, a Higher National Diploma (HND) or undergraduate degree. For these types of programmes, typically described as vocational studies and aimed at the helping professions, you may well be returning to study as an adult. Consequently, it may be quite some time since you were last in formal study and this might be anxiety-provoking! Equally, you might be working in the field of health and social care and be sponsored by your employer to gain a qualification or perhaps you are an experienced practitioner keen to expand your knowledge and understanding in this field through a formal qualification. Regardless of your circumstances, undertaking study at a higher education level and becoming a student can be a challenging process. As you begin this new aspect of your life, this book will introduce you to some key ideas and skills for study and to provide the foundation for a productive and successful time at college or university.

This book is intended to support you in your studies by helping you to think about the transition to college and university, providing you with the skills to support you in your learning whilst there, and learning in practice or on practice placements. Developing these learning skills will also enhance your motivation in your studies. As you begin to appreciate why these study skills are so important in your programme of study, your desire to succeed, to persist and to achieve a successful outcome will be increased.

The idea of being motivated in your learning is an important one: as mentioned earlier, returning to study can be a challenge, particularly as you have to make adjustments to your life to manage your studies. In addition, when you go out on your placements you will be judged by the quality of your work; you will have to demonstrate your competence in relation to meeting practice requirements set by the course, and, equally, work that you produce in college or university will be assessed according to set criteria. The fact you are now being judged in relation to these factors can be anxiety-provoking precisely because these decisions matter in relation to your sense of achievement, esteem and future career plans.

What has felt familiar – things that you have done in your job, indeed, your ability to do the job – now becomes something that can be looked at and questioned in different ways. This is also the case when producing work for academic purposes: writing, for example, can now be a very different experience. In addition, your new studies are likely to make demands on your private life; you have to learn to manage your time in different ways in order to meet deadlines set by the course and to maintain your relationships with family and friends. New learning experiences may make you begin to see yourself, your life and your work in new ways that can be exciting but also daunting. Other people too may start to see a change in you and this can cause your relationship with these people to alter. Considering all of these issues, returning to formal studying is not necessarily as straightforward as it may at first feel. Therefore, your commitment to your studies and motivation to persist are important.

Regardless of your motive or reason for studying, one key thing we are sure you will want is to be successful in your studies. This requires you to believe that you are capable and have the potential to succeed. In committing yourself to your new learning, you must see the learning experience as having value and have an expectation that you are likely to succeed. The concept of self-efficacy, the belief in yourself as able to learn, understand and be successful, is crucial to your approach to learning and your motivation. This book aims to support you in achieving your potential and being successful in your new studies.

As the title of this book suggests, learning to study makes use of certain skills that are effective in helping you to be successful. So 'study skills' suggest that there are a number of approaches and qualities that can be developed to enhance your understanding and abilities and consequently support you in your learning. For example, a key part of the learning process at higher education level is that you are able to reflect on your learning experiences to show evidence of understanding and that you are also able to transfer your understanding to practice. This is typically expressed as your ability to translate theory into practice; that is, to see the connections between what you have learnt at university and apply this understanding in practice, or in a work setting. The ability to be reflective as a key part of being successful in your studies is covered in this book through reading and practical activities.

Indeed, throughout the book we have included activities and reflection points which will help you practise some of the skills we highlight. Learning is presented as both a cognitive activity and an active process. Importantly, the reflection points provide opportunities for you to pause in your reading and begin the process of attempting to make sense of the learning material by thinking about the issues discussed. Together, the activities and reflection points will help you to engage with what you read and encourage your skills as an active learner. The process involves you being able to understand why and how learning happens. They will help you to be successful in your studies and practice placements.

Chapter 1 requires readers to think about the transition to higher education. It introduces the type of learning that is encouraged at college and university. Specifically, students are expected to acquire a 'deep approach' to their learning, thinking about what they are learning and taking an active approach to making sense of the new learning material. There is an expectation that, as you progress through your studies, you take increasing responsibility for your learning by undertaking guided private study to enhance your understanding. Activities are used to support you in making sense of the new material. You are aiming for long-term retention and understanding of new information. The material in this chapter will help you to begin to see how a deep approach enables you to make better sense of your new subject and apply new learning in a practice setting.

Chapter 2 considers the importance of interpersonal communication skills, particularly focusing on verbal and non-verbal communication and listening skills. These are crucial in your studies but are also important in working with people in your professional role. The chapter aims to raise your awareness of these skills, which are often taken for granted with little consideration for the consequences. The activities in this chapter will raise your awareness of the process of interpretation and increase your verbal skills by expanding your vocabulary. This is essential in your professional role so that you are able to communicate effectively and purposively with colleagues and people you work with, as well as being essential in your studies so that you can meet the requirements of your academic work.

Chapters 3 and 4 continue the theme of developing the skills of communication. Chapter 3 is divided into two parts, with the first half concentrating on developing competence in information and communication technology (ICT). Good use of ICT is central to helping you develop confidence in finding relevant books and articles necessary for your studies. Subsequently, there are skills necessary for judging the relevance and validity of the literature you are considering. Part two moves on to the importance of developing reading and writing skills, with some emphasis on essay writing in order to help you produce work of a suitable standard for the assessed requirements of your course.

The importance of presentation skills is discussed in Chapter 4. Presentation skills are commonly required as part of your studies and are a key skill in professional practice. Therefore, good planning, preparation and practice are necessary and the chapter is packed with activities designed to help you practise and enhance your abilities in these areas.

Opportunities for practice learning are a key part of professional programmes for people studying towards a qualification in the helping professions. In Chapter 5 we emphasise the importance of practice learning opportunities to assess your competence in relation to the knowledge, skills and values associated with your professional programme of study. Placements provide a key opportunity for you to demonstrate your understanding of your academic learning and its application to practice and your continuing professional development.

The final chapter explores the importance of reflection as an aid to developing understanding and enhancing your learning. The term 'reflective practitioner' is relevant both in your academic studies and as part of developing your professional role in practice. Courses commonly require you to produce an assessed piece of reflective writing and Chapter 6 also considers different models of reflection with a view to developing your reflective capacity and reflective writing skills.

Each chapter ends with a summary highlighting the key points of the chapter as well as further reading to encourage you to widen your understanding. A useful glossary of terms is also included, providing succinct definitions of some of the key terms used throughout the book and by colleges and universities. The glossary will support you in making a successful transition to your degree studies.

Undertaking a degree in the helping professions can be a rewarding experience but it can also be a challenge – you are in a new environment and from early on you need to meet the demands of the course. However, if you have been successful in gaining a place on a degree course, then you should believe that you have the potential to be successful in your studies. This book will support and help develop the key skills that you need in order to be successful. Engaging with the many practical exercises will help you avoid the pitfalls of a limited approach to your studies. Reading and engaging with the exercises will mean that you are well prepared for what lies ahead and, as a result, you will be giving yourself the best opportunity to be successful in your studies.

1 LEARNING TO LEARN

CHAPTER OBJECTIVES

By the end of this chapter you should be able to:

- understand what is meant by learning and that it is concerned with an active process of meaning-making and understanding;

- understand and identify the difference between 'deep' and 'surface' approaches to learning;

- recognise a variety of approaches you can adopt in taking an active approach to your programme of study and manage the learning in ways that promote a 'deep' approach to learning.

Introduction

This opening chapter can be read as a kind of 'scene setter', preparing you to think about your studies as you embark on your new programme. It will help you to think generally about what is meant by learning and study and prepare you for your learning at university or college. This is important because your course provider makes an important judgment about the quality of your learning, which is a powerful moulder of how you learn. You can view this chapter as providing an insider's guide to helping you successfully manage the learning environment of higher education in ways that allow you to achieve your goal of completing your qualification in health or social care.

What is learning?

First, think about how you would define learning. Complete Activity 1.1.

ACTIVITY 1.1

Spend a few minutes completing this exercise.

• How would you define learning?

Jot down a couple of sentences or key terms that you feel describe what learning is.

Comment

One of the first things that come to mind is the idea that learning is about acquiring new ideas and information and making sense of the material. The process of making sense suggests an engagement with that information for a purpose. Implicitly, this indicates that the learning is meaningful for us: we want to learn (regardless of different motivations) and therefore it has some use or purpose for us.

In thinking about what is learning, you may have thought about a particular activity, for instance, swimming or learning to ride a bike, and maybe can see some parallels with our description above.

Experiences like learning to ride a bike conjure up thoughts of learning as an activity that has purpose and also bring to mind ideas about motivation. Thinking about practical activities as examples of learning also captures the idea that learning is an active process of doing. So, learning to swim, ride a bike, cook or drive a car involves practice. This is suggestive of learning as a skill – learning something new and practising until we have reached a level of competency. The goal is to acquire an ability whereby we no longer consider our learning as a new skill but rather, it is a skill in which we are proficient and which we can perform independently.

A focus on learning as a practical activity suggests a view of learning as a product or outcome of behaviour and is most recognisable in the form of new behaviour. Whilst this outcome approach is important in terms of describing learning, it can be challenged. For instance, do we always need to perform (i.e. do something) for learning to take place? And does our behaviour always change because we have learnt something? Also, describing learning simply as a product or outcome limits the potential for change. So, for instance, we might reflect back on previous experience and consider how we might change our behaviour in the future. This suggests the potential for learning from an event, so we are not only learning to do (as in the outcome approach) but we are also learning how.

'Learning how' highlights that learning is also a process. This approach is also suggested in our view of learning (Activity 1.1). When we talk about learning as acquiring new ideas and information, it requires the process of engagement with the new material for it to make sense or, in other words, to mean something to us. So, in attaining new knowledge of something, we are learning how to make sense of it. Learning therefore becomes a process of meaning-making.

Importantly, our learning affects us as we engage in the process, since it is we who are meaning-making and looking to make sense of the new material. So in this context, learning is both an active and a cognitive process, as in doing and questioning the new material for it to make sense. Since we are striving for meaning in our learning, we can also consider that an important component to learning is our level of motivation towards the process or the new material. This applies to whether we are learning for pleasure or where we have an academic or professional goal in mind, such as wanting to become a childcare worker, nurse or teacher.

Perhaps now we can begin to see some of the key constituent parts of a description of learning.

- Learning represents a process of knowledge acquisition through a cognitive process of active engagement with the new learning material in order for it to make sense and to develop our understanding.
- Learning is a cumulative process that builds upon previous learning to enhance and develop our understanding.

This new learning can also be considered as 'portable knowledge': we carry this new understanding around with us and are able to begin applying this new understanding to new and less familiar contexts, thus developing a more enhanced understanding. The idea that learning is cumulative suggests a process of building or constructing new understanding and that knowledge can be manipulated and applied to new experiences, consequently enhancing our understanding of the social world. However, this cognitive journey of building up our understanding is not necessarily unproblematic or, indeed, linear. We may learn something that conflicts with our previous understanding or indeed our beliefs, which makes the new material difficult to engage with and drives us on to be more critical in our understanding. Ultimately we can describe learning as a process of meaning-making that enhances or even transforms our understanding. By striving for understanding and engaging in this cognitive process of making sense, we engage in the critical process of meaning-making.

Fry et al. (2001) describe learning as being about how we perceive and make sense of the world.

> *It can be about abstract principles, factual information, the acquisition of methods, techniques and approaches, about ideas, behaviour appropriate to types of situations, recognition, and finally, about reasoning.*
>
> (Fry et al., 2001, p21)

All of these different factors can be taken by learners as representing 'new material' with which they can engage in order to make sense and apply this new knowledge in relevant contexts.

Student approaches to learning

So far, we have considered defining what is meant by learning and asked you to describe what learning means to you. In higher education, the field in which universities are situated, there has been much research into student learning; however this does not necessarily translate into a straightforward picture of how to inform teaching. This is because there are many variables to consider. For instance: the student population is diverse, not only in terms of age, but also in previous educational experience, social background and the expectations that students bring to the university environment. In particular, there are differences in how we approach the new learning we encounter in class. Individual learners will use a variety of different methods in their approach to learning and, of course, there are differences in subject knowledge that alter how we approach the learning task.

Ramsden (2003, p23) suggests that, as students progress through higher education, they develop increasingly sophisticated ways of thinking, typically progressing from a 'lower level', where they conceive of knowledge as *conveniently packaged and static facts and techniques. Learning these packages implies gaining authoritative information about them* (Ramsden, 2003, p26). At this lower level, learning is perceived to be about memory and accurate recall. This is described as an *absolutistic view of knowledge and learning,* but a more sophisticated way of thinking about learning is described as representing a *relativistic conception.* At this higher level:

> *knowledge is then seen to be uncertain; the truth always remains provisional . . . students will have learned to commit themselves to personal values and particular interpretations of evidence, while at the same time acknowledging the existence of alternative interpretations of 'reality' and being capable of continuing to learn.*

(Ramsden, 2003, p27)

Key concept

Defining learning

Saljo (1979, cited in Ramsden, 2003) conducted an interview study with students, asking them to describe their view of learning. From their replies, he identified five different categories of learning.

1. Learning as a quantitative increase in knowledge. Learning is acquiring information or 'knowing a lot'.
2. Learning is memorising. Learning is storing information that can be reproduced.
3. Learning is acquiring facts, skills and methods that can be retained and used as necessary.
4. Learning is making sense or abstracting meaning. Learning involves relating parts of the subject matter to each other and the real world.
5. Learning as interpreting and understanding reality in a different way. Learning involves comprehending the world by reinterpreting knowledge.

(Ramsden, 2003, p28)

(Saljo's classification is hierarchical, that is, each conception implies all the rest beneath it.)

What we can deduce so far is that within higher education there are expectations that, as you progress through your studies, you will develop a more critical approach to learning and understanding. This is one that moves away from 'the teacher as knowing' with reliance on memorisation and accurate recall to a more sophisticated approach that requires you to engage actively in your learning in order to promote meaning and critical understanding and generate new knowledge. This view of learning fits in with definitions 4 and 5 above in the Key concept box.

So what can you do to prepare yourself for learning at higher education level that promotes this more sophisticated approach?

Preparing to study

When we talk about studying, we are talking about the way in which *teaching and learning is organised in formal programmes of study* (Burns and Sinfield, 2003, p15). So studying is the course work you do in order to pass your degree programme. Study skills can be described as the range of techniques that you can develop to help you manage your studies successfully.

The way in which *teaching and learning is organised* suggests a relationship between the two. Marton and Saljo (1997) is a good example of research that shows the relationship between how students learn and how this is affected by teaching. Their research points out that students adopt different learning approaches according to how they see the learning task, that is, their perception of what is expected from a learning activity such as an essay or presentation. Different approaches to learning can determine the extent to which students engage in their learning and ultimately, of course, the quality of the outcome, that is, how well they do in the learning activity. This suggests that there are more productive and less productive ways of learning: these different approaches can be described as either 'deep' approaches to learning or 'surface' approaches. When thinking about how you approach your learning, you need to be aware of which approach you are adopting.

Deep and surface approaches to learning

When we talk about deep approaches to learning, we are thinking about our definition of learning that emphasises learning as a cognitive (i.e. thinking) process of engaging with the learning material in order to make sense and understand. New learning builds upon previous understanding so that we gain a fuller picture or a more all-round conception of the subject. Deep or meaningful learning is concerned with trying to understand the whole picture – so, we might think, *how does this new information fit in with what I already know and help me make better sense of the whole picture?* Through a process of critical engagement and analysis of the new information, we try to see how this new information links with what is already known. Overall, we are building up a fuller picture that leads to a better understanding that, in turn, is likely to lead to greater long-term retention of the new information. This new understanding can then be used in new, less familiar contexts. Deep learning is about understanding the subject material and promoting long-term retention of the information so that it can be applied in the 'real world'. It represents an active approach to you managing your learning coupled with a motivation to understand the subject.

In contrast, surface or superficial learning concentrates more on the 'here and now'. This approach tends to promote rote learning or the memorisation of key facts and fails to link the new material to the wider picture. Adopting this approach, surface learners tend to concentrate on what they think the teacher wants them to know. If you like, this can been seen as 'learning for the teacher' rather than for yourself.

The new learning material is simply accepted – *this is what I need to know*. New learning becomes a series of unrelated information and is an approach to learning that yields only superficial retention of information that fails to promote understanding or long-term retention of the information.

CASE STUDY 1.1

Anna is a first-year student on a foundation degree in health and social care. She has worked for several years as a social care assistant for a large independent care agency providing home care support to vulnerable adults living in the community. She is being sponsored by her employer to complete her degree after successfully completing an in-house National Vocational Qualification (NVQ) at level 3 the year before.

During her classes, Anna made copious notes, often asking the tutor to repeat what had been said so that she could write it down correctly. In one of her modules, Human Growth and Development (HGD), the class was reviewing the importance of making professional judgments about 'what the matter is' based upon students' knowledge of HGD and the issues presented to them. The class was working in small groups completing a case study where they had to identify 'what the matter is' and which theory of human growth and development they felt best helped them make sense of the case study. As they progressed through the module, the class also looked at different ways of supporting vulnerable children and adults and the range of professionals and provision of services that could support the client. They had to make links between theories of HGD, using this to inform their judgments and decide what support and services could be drawn upon.

For the end-of-module assignment, the class had to complete a similar exercise. They had a case study and the assignment criteria identified what they had to do. In particular, they were asked to consider one theory of HGD, to describe it and then explain how it was useful in helping them to identify what the issues were in the case study. They then had to consider how professional services or interventions could help minimise problems or provide for effective support.

When Anna began working on her assignment, she looked back at her lecture notes and used them as the basis for completing her assignment. She wrote generally about all the theories of HGD and identified a wide range of issues that she felt were important and needed to be addressed before exploring what interventions could be used.

Unfortunately, Anna was unsuccessful in her assignment. In the feedback supplied by the module tutor it was identified that her work was too general and did not address specifically the assignment criteria. In identifying all the theories of human growth and development, Anna's understanding lacked depth and was too general, since she had not applied a particular theory to the case study. In failing to identify one theory, Anna had missed an important opportunity to demonstrate her understanding of this approach in depth and consequently failed to identify those factors in the case that could be interpreted from a particular perspective of HGD. Her assessment was too general, with too many issues identified that represented the whole spectrum of theories of HGD. Her view about 'what the matter is' represented a 'scattergun' approach to identifying all the factors that Anna felt warranted attention. As a result, the case was overwhelmed by a number of interventions that demonstrated a lack of understanding and focus on the relevant issues and failed to identify an intervention that could most usefully support the client. Overall, the work was largely unstructured and too general, lacking coherence between all these interconnecting factors. Anna had failed to realise that the module had provided her with a framework for making sense of the range of difficulties that clients may face and present to professionals working with them. In order to 'make sense', Anna had to 'see' the connection between HGD theories and how these inform our view of what the matter is, particularly that there should be a relationship between this and interventions that, at best, result in a positive and meaningful outcome for the client.

Comment

From reading Anna's case study, you can begin to identify some of the characteristics of a surface and deep approach to learning.

- Anna relied too heavily on lecture notes. In class she concentrated so hard on taking down all the lecturer said that she failed to listen and engage properly with the content. She was more concerned with having a full set of lecture notes than with understanding what was actually said. In her assignment, she mainly reproduced these lecture notes, with little evidence of understanding, or that she had made use of recommended texts to supplement her understanding.
- In class work, Anna preferred to sit quietly and not engage in group work discussion. Instead, she waited for feedback from the group and for the lecturer to identify 'the right answer' rather than actively participating by engaging and questioning the learning material to try and make sense.
- Anna had difficulty seeing how the module fitted together – she could not see the whole picture. Instead she took the different subject areas as separate and unrelated and had difficulty identifying the relationship between how theories of HGD aid our judgment about 'what the matter is' and what interventions should be used. Instead Anna felt that what was needed was to learn all these areas as separate and reproduce them with little understanding of how they fitted together.
- Anna had trouble making links between the different subject areas of the module and failed to relate new material to what had been taught before. For the end-of-module assignment, Anna felt that all she had to do was reproduce material from the lectures and present it as 'everything I know from this module' rather than appreciating what the assignment was asking for and using her knowledge selectively to demonstrate her understanding.

If learning is about making sense and understanding, then we can see that overly relying on surface approaches to learning is not effective. It means we limit the possibilities for understanding and being able to use this new material. If we are unable to use this new material, then we have difficulty in applying the new information in meaningful ways that make sense and that can be usefully applied. In Anna's example, undertaking a degree is not just about learning an academic subject. Health and social care is also an applied activity – you will go out on placement, and you will be expected to use your understanding in meaningful ways in order to demonstrate your understanding of the process of care work.

Promoting a deep approach to learning

So what can you do to improve your chances of success in your studies? Although Anna's case study provides an example of a surface approach to learning and the common result of a poor outcome in an assignment, it is important to remember that deep or surface approaches to learning are just that – they are approaches and not in themselves characteristics of individual learners. In other words, we can adopt both approaches in our learning, but being overly reliant on surface approaches is likely to lead to an unsatisfactory experience of learning.

What can you learn from Anna's example and what can you do to benefit most from your studies? In the earlier section on preparing to study, we identified the relationship between teaching and learning – in other words, how you are taught can affect the approach you take to learning. It is important to recognise this because how your programme of study is taught can affect how successful you are in your studies. Being aware of the different teaching and learning strategies used in your programme of study means that you can take a more active approach towards your learning – you will be taking more responsibility about how you manage your studies.

In the next section we will identify important factors for you to consider when identifying your course and emphasise again the importance of motivation. We will move on to discuss a range of teaching and learning strategies and how you can benefit from them by adopting a deeper approach to learning.

Thinking about your course of study

At this stage, you may have already begun a programme of study in the helping professions, or you may be thinking of applying to a university or college to study. Either way, one of the first things to remember is the importance of your motivation to study. Since you know that learning is about making sense of new material and engaging in a process of meaning-making and understanding, you can see that successful learning requires an active engagement in the learning process. Therefore, it is important to be clear about your reasons for studying and the level of interest you have in the subject matter. You should remember that learning something new is hindered if your level of interest in the subject is poor – you are not likely to be inspired to engage in your studies if you are not interested.

ACTIVITY 1.3
Write down your replies to the following questions.

- What are your reasons for wanting to study your subject of interest?
- What is your end goal? What do you want to achieve?
- How would you describe your motivation towards this goal?
- How can you maintain a good level of motivation in your studies?
- What characteristics do you have that can help you maintain your motivation?
- Can you call on other people/support structures to help you in maintaining a commitment towards your studies?

In thinking about your commitment to studying for a degree and your level of motivation, it is helpful to have made enquiries about a programme of study you are interested in. You can, for instance, check out a university or college prospectus, read about the course content and what subject areas are covered (i.e. the curriculum) and gain knowledge of the entry requirements for the course.

Increasingly, colleges and universities offer open or 'taster' days – opportunities for prospective students to come along to the university and listen to talks about the range of available courses. These open days provide a good opportunity for you to see the learning environment for yourself (they often provide campus tours for you to see the range of facilities available). They allow you to get 'a feel for the place' and make a more informed decision that this is an environment you feel comfortable studying in. In addition, subject-specific talks, in Anna's case about the foundation degree in health and social care, will introduce you to the course curriculum and provide examples of how you will be taught (that is, the learning and teaching strategies). They give you a more informed view about health and social care, alongside details of the selection process (meeting the entry requirements, applying to the university, what happens at interview and what the interview panel is looking for).

Thinking back to your replies to the questions in Activity 1.3, how active have you been in researching your programme of study?

Once you have been accepted on the course, there is a process of induction – the formal process of introducing you to the course and the wider university or college. Often this will involve introductions to key sections in the university, for instance, student support services, which provide information and advice on a range of non-academic issues, such as student finance, counselling and welfare services, academic skills support and an introduction to the library and computing services.

In addition, induction is the time when you formally enrol and register on the course and become a student of the university. It is worth remembering that induction and enrolment are extremely important. At this early stage in your programme, the level of information you will be faced with can seem overwhelming. You are likely to have to complete a number of different forms (for registration and enrolment purposes, either online or manually) and be provided with lots of verbal information and reading material, for instance, a programme handbook and other student guides. Because the level of information is so high, many students just 'go with the flow', finding much of the information difficult to retain simply because there is so much of it.

You are in a new environment with new people, the experience seems unfamiliar and in some cases can be anxiety-provoking. Don't worry – this is a common feeling! In the first few days of the induction process, it can feel more like an administrative task of completing lots of paperwork, listening and collecting lots of information, so bring a bag. However, induction is very important and you need to attend your course's induction programme – it's where you begin to make friends, you will retain some of the information and you will start to become familiar with the environment. Importantly, a good induction programme will begin to establish a specific course identity, helping you reach a view that the programme of study on which you have enrolled is the degree you want to study. It is also an important opportunity to meet members of the teaching staff at a more informal level before the teaching starts. This can all begin to add to a positive sense that you 'fit in' and have made the right decision to come and study.

Vocational qualifications, such as foundation degrees or Higher National Diplomas (HNDs), can attract more 'non-traditional' applicants – so rather than being a typical college or university group, this group can include people who are embarking on the course as a second career, people with family or caring responsibilities, individuals who have been out of education for some time and those with a variety of qualifications, such as NVQs and Council for Awards in Care, Health and Education (CACHE) diplomas. Others may call on their life and work experience as a means of gaining entry to the course. For these reasons you may find yourself on a course where some of your classmates are focused more on obtaining the qualification than on being part of a wider student community and, if you like, enjoying the student life.

Whether you see yourself as more focused on the course or enjoying the wider benefits of student life, if you are committed to your studies, you still need to find ways of managing your time effectively in order to complete your studies. Time management is an important skill to cultivate. Life still goes on when you start university, and family, friends, relationships and work commitments need to managed and worked on alongside managing the work requirements of your course. So, thinking back to your responses to Activity 1.3, what levels of support do you have as you begin your studies and how prepared are your family and friends for what is involved in studying for a degree?

What can be described as the 'first-year experience' is very important and the first few weeks of your course should contribute towards a positive outlook for the rest of your studies. The first year is commonly described as a 'foundation' year where you study core modules (i.e. all students complete these modules – there are no option choices available). These core modules introduce you to a range of subjects that contribute towards an understanding about the role of health and social care or early years and childhood studies in society and the roles and responsibilities of professionals working in that field – together they form the basis on which you will build your understanding of the subject. The first year should help to establish your curiosity in the subject, making efforts to engage you in learning activities and engendering a feeling in you to do well. You should make an active commitment towards making use of the university support structures that are in place to support you in your learning and the support from tutors and formal learning opportunities to engage with other students, such as through course-related group work.

If you are unsure about a module, don't be shy about seeking out the module leader for further information and support, or using tutorials to help you in your learning tasks. Personal tutors are there to help you if you have any concerns that may have an impact on your studies. In seeking a positive first-year experience, universities and colleges want you to succeed – that is why the student support services are in place for you. It is worth bearing a simple fact in mind – universities don't want you to fail in your studies any more than you do. Universities have a high commitment towards supporting student retention – that is, making sure that students have the support they need in order to succeed in their studies.

So far we have discussed generally cultivating an interest in your chosen programme of study – from initial enquiry to induction and the notion of the first-year experience. A willingness to be informed, knowledge of the components of these early experiences and making use of the support structures should lay the groundwork for a positive first-year experience. Remind yourself again of your answers to Activity 1.3 and your level of motivation to engage in the subject matter of your degree. In the final section of this chapter, we will consider what you can expect from your classroom experiences.

Now that I am on the course

We are now considering what is described as learning and teaching strategies – the range of learning activities that you might be expected to undertake in your learning and understanding of your programme of study. At this point, you should remember the relationship between approaches to learning and the learning task you are engaged with and that 'deep' approaches to learning require an active engagement with the learning material in order to make sense and understand.

As part of good practice, module leaders (those who teach you specific subjects) should provide you with a copy of the module guide. This details what is covered in the module, the types of assessment involved and a recommended reading list or further learning resources. Module guides are important because they provide you with key information about what the module is about, that is, the module aims, and what you can expect to learn (learning outcomes). The learning outcomes indicate what you can expect to know at the end of the module and are used as the basis of assessment. In addition, module guides point out what you will be studying in the module (the indicative content or module curriculum).

In learning something new, formal programmes of study such as university courses expect you to demonstrate your understanding of this new material and you should not be surprised to know that in order to pass a module, you will be expected to undertake an assessment of your learning. Assessment allows you to demonstrate your knowledge, understanding and abilities in using the subject matter. Again, a module guide should provide you with details about the module assessment and the assessment criteria, that is, what areas of understanding should be demonstrated in your assessment. And here is another fact that is worth remembering – assessments are not designed to test you on what you have not covered in the module. As stated above, the assessment is linked to the module learning outcomes and the relationship between the assessment and the learning outcomes should be transparent to you. Put simply, your assessment (what you are expected to do in order to demonstrate your understanding and abilities) will relate directly to what you have been learning about – the learning outcomes.

Early in their studies many students are typically motivated in their learning towards the assessment – in other words, the assessment drives your learning. The danger with this is that a surface approach to learning can develop. So in class, to support you in moving towards a deep learning approach, a variety of learning activities are used, for example, group work, working on case studies or doing presentations. This variety is used to enable you to think about and process information in different contexts and to use a range of skills to support your learning. Overall, these learning activities help you make sense of what you have been taught, so that when it comes to your assessment you can draw on your own abilities developed in class to allow you to demonstrate your understanding.

You should see again here the importance of an active approach to study that encourages deep or meaningful learning. The range of learning activities that are in use has been developed to support you. They embrace different learning styles so that all students have equally as much opportunity to benefit from their experience. Programmes will make use of a number of different learning and teaching strategies, such as:

- seminars (where you are expected to have undertaken some recommended reading or a learning task in preparation);
- case studies;
- principles of problem-based learning;
- group work;
- lectures;
- practice learning opportunities, i.e. placements;
- presentations;
- role-plays;
- computer-assisted learning;
- service user and carer involvement;
- guided private study.

The above list provides an example of the range of strategies that may be adopted to support and encourage you in your learning and understanding. So, for instance, group work gives you the opportunity to discuss with peers some of the ideas that have been presented in the class. It also develops your abilities to work with other people. Discussions allow you to test your understanding, debate, clarify or share your understanding, and, in turn, learn from others. Case studies allow you to think about practice and application of the knowledge you have acquired, and role-plays allow you the opportunity to develop and practise skills in working with others. Such 'acting-out' activities allow you 'to see' and practise what you have been learning.

Your programme of study is not only an academic subject but also an applied activity that requires practice to cultivate. It is important that you engage with these learning activities and do not adopt a passive approach to learning, as in Anna's case example. There may well be right answers in particular cases or more effective ways of applying your knowledge or understanding, but the classroom is an ideal and safe environment in which to practise and begin to apply your understanding, and to receive the constructive feedback that contributes towards a more enhanced understanding.

Feedback provides an important function in your learning, whether it is feedback from your peers or from the module tutor, as it should contribute towards developing your understanding. This should remind you of a main focus of this book, that is, the potential for change from learning. Feedback provides you with an opportunity to reflect on what you have done and how you can enhance your learning in order to develop a better understanding. We can learn from our experiences (in this case, learning from class-based activities that we have undertaken) and use the feedback to think forward – that is, if I did this again, what could I do differently to improve it? Even if what we have done is good, and the feedback is positive, we should still be able to learn from the experience and apply it in new contexts in the future.

In addition, try not to think of feedback as only summative involving formal feedback at the end of the module following an assessment. Feedback should represent *a continuous loop* (Hounsell, 2007) and good teachers make use of formative feedback throughout their module. For feedback to be useful it should indicate what you can do to improve your understanding, as well as identifying what has been done well. The student who adopts deep approaches to learning will use feedback to look forward and consider what can be done to enhance performance and understanding. Both types of feedback, formative during the class and summative following an assessment, allow you to pace your learning. Feedback provides an opportunity for you to reflect on your approach to study, gauge your understanding, plan and take an active role in managing your learning.

> **REFLECTION POINT**
> Review the discussion about deep learning and draw up a list of factors that you think are important in developing a deep approach to learning.

CHAPTER SUMMARY

- Learning is a cognitive process of active engagement with new material that builds upon what has previously been learnt, in order to enhance and develop your understanding.
- In higher education, learning is associated with conceptual change and development that involves *comprehending the world by reinterpreting knowledge* (Saljo, 1979, cited in Ramsden, 2003, p28).
- You should aim to develop a 'deep' approach to learning as this is most likely to yield success in your studies, contribute towards a positive first-year experience and see you returning to complete your studies.
- Learning is an active process of engagement: you are a key player in your education and you should think carefully about your motivation to study and embark on a professional or vocational programme of study.

The next chapter concentrates on verbal and non-verbal communication skills which are necessary for passing both your course and your practice placement.

FURTHER READING

Adams, R (ed) (2007) *Foundations of Health and Social Care*. Basingstoke: Palgrave Macmillan.
This comprehensive book is aimed at foundation degree students covering key theories and practice skills in health and social care.

Burns, T and Sinfield, S (2012) *Essential Study Skills* (3rd edition). London: Sage.
This popular study skills text is aimed at university students and provides generic coverage of skill development to support students across any degree programme.

2 VERBAL AND NON-VERBAL COMMUNICATION SKILLS

CHAPTER OBJECTIVES

By the end of this chapter you should be able to:

- understand the difference between non-verbal and verbal communication;
- appreciate the importance of active listening;
- realise the importance of developing a varied and effective lexicon.

Together, these points contribute towards achieving positive outcomes both in your studies and for the people you will work with as part of your professional practice.

Introduction

College and university are about much more than the inevitable essays, presentations or exams that assess your knowledge, understanding and skills; however, it is this aspect that exercises students the most. This and the following chapters begin to explore a range of important communication skills that are necessary as part of your academic and professional development. In this chapter we concentrate on verbal and non-verbal communication skills, including the skill of active listening, whilst the following two chapters consider further the wide-ranging nature of communication. Chapter 3 considers how your communication skills are supported by skills in the effective use of information and communication technology (ICT) and Chapter 4 focuses on presentational skills.

Key concept

Communication

Non-verbal communication is defined in this chapter as anything other than words or utterances that are used to convey a message or meaning. This involves body language, including posture, gestures and expressions, and even how you dress. Since first impressions count, non-verbal communication perhaps most profoundly demonstrates the importance of good communication in our everyday lives. Our emotions are expressed through non-verbal communication in our facial expressions or gestures. How we are seen by and how we see others are subject to interpretation as part of the process of understanding what is being communicated. So we may look at a young person dressed in a certain way and her accompanying gestures and label her as 'Emo' or 'Goth', but what does this really tell us about that young person's life and experience? It is important that we seek clarity and check our assumptions and interpretations of body language.

Verbal communication includes words and utterances. We convey meaning through pitch, tone of voice, volume and speed of speech or noises. In writing words we emphasise by using **bold**, *italics*, underlining or CAPITALS or a combination of these: <u>**EMPHASIS**</u>. Significantly, words themselves do not always communicate meaning: the word 'afraid' does not impart fear. That comes in part through the sound and emotion used in expressing the word. Consequently it is important that you hear what is said and how it is said. Good verbal and written communication is dependent on the development of good listening skills and an appropriate and effective lexicon, that is, vocabulary and understanding of words. Emotion can also be expressed in written form through adjectives and adverbs or symbols such as emoticons: :).

Active listening is often expressed as an essential part of effective communication in professional practice. The word 'active' is used to emphasise that effective listening is a *mental activity that requires effort and concentration* (Williams, 1997, p47). When you are concentrating on the purpose of a tutorial and engaging with the tutor to impart or elicit information, you are not passive in the process. Both your verbal and non-verbal responses show the tutor that you understand and are engaged in the conversation, and vice versa.

Understanding the importance of communication skills

The report of the National Committee of Inquiry into Higher Education (the Dearing Report, 1998) brought into focus the skills necessary for student success whatever your programme of study and intended profession. The report highlighted four essential attributes for study and later employment: (1) communication skills; (2) numeracy; (3) ICT; and (4) learning how to learn. This message has been reiterated many times since, particularly by employers. Communication skills include verbal, written, presentational, non-verbal, individual and group skills.

As a result these skills are used within module specifications to define the assessment outcomes for your studies and, importantly, a successful outcome is not just about what you know but also about how you communicate this. This is demonstrated in the way that assessment outcomes are written in the module specifications for your course. Examples are given in the box overleaf.

Knowledge and understanding

This is about what you know, such as:

- theories and methods of intervention with a child, young person and family;
- the nature and context of complex practice with people.

Cognitive and intellectual skills

This refers to how you use the knowledge that you have, usually expressed using a key verb, such as: understand, describe, analyse, critically analyse, evaluate, synthesise. The particular verb used will depend on your year of study. In year one you might describe or analyse; in your second year you might be expected to critically analyse, and in your final year you could be required to evaluate and synthesise. These are written like this:

- Describe and analyse data/evidence from a range of sources.
- Critically analyse the key theories and methods of intervention.

Practical and professional skills

The key skills required for your particular course or future occupation, for example, reflection or work with other professionals. These can also be accompanied by one of the verbs mentioned above. Examples include the following.

- Critically reflect upon experience in placement of work with patients or service users.
- Describe the context of interprofessional collaboration.

Key transferable skills

Other skills are useful in a range of contexts and for a range of purposes both for your studies and later for your work. Typically these include an ability to find and use a range of information and to present it appropriately depending on context. Examples include the following.

- Use IT equipment to research, write, present papers and to discuss issues with peers.
- Gather, review and manage information.
- Work effectively as a member of a study group.

As you can see, three of the four groups of assessment outcomes specifically mention skills and this and the following chapters will help you to identify and enhance the range of skills necessary for a successful outcome in your studies and work.

The rules of communication

The centrality of communication cannot be overestimated since human beings constantly communicate – it is what makes us inherently social. However, this involves us understanding and adhering to a set of rules to which we give little conscious thought. Reports and letters follow certain expectations. Moreover, think about the times you have been put off by someone who has poor communication skills: perhaps the person mumbles, doesn't hold eye contact or gets too close. Indeed, we only really become aware of our own communication behaviour when someone else acts outside the norm. A challenge for you is to develop your awareness of the rules of communication since not to do so could place you in an awkward situation.

At the foundation of the rules of communication you should bear in mind that *communication is by definition interactive and always takes place within a relationship* and *communication is context-related* (Koprowska, 2005, p6). This has wide implications for your studies and professional practice since you need to be aware that you will be communicating with a wide range of people with a variety of needs and expectations: tutors, peers, placement mentors or practice teachers, children, young people, service users and patients, for example. In understanding the needs of the people with whom you communicate, you will realise that the range of situations involved requires use of a variety of media, such as a written essay or an individual poster presentation for your tutor, a group presentation to the rest of your class, a report or assessment for your mentor and play with a child. There is a complex relationship between your knowledge of the people involved and the communication skills required to meet those needs successfully.

Remember, an appropriate rule with one person or in one context may not apply with another person or in a different context. A hand-written essay with lots of crossings out is unlikely to meet the requirements for academic assessment; verbal communication may be inappropriate for a person who is hearing-impaired or deaf; eye contact is not respectful in some cultures and a sign or gesture may mean something completely different for some people. In order to ensure better outcomes for you and those with whom you work, it is important that you constantly rise to the challenge of recognising the relationship and interaction in which the communication is based and the context of that relationship. Understanding the range of cultural norms, rules and conventions will help to project understanding, competence and respect.

ACTIVITY 2.1

Without drawing attention to yourself, observe the communication behaviour of five different people. Make a note of the following:

- What do you notice about how they communicate?
- Are there key similarities or differences in their communication?
- What rules might be governing their communication?
- Which of these rules govern how you communicate?

We will return to your observations in a later activity.

Being able to use communication skills in ways which are fit for purpose, that is, ways that are appropriate to the task and context, is essential for developing confidence and achieving good outcomes in your studies as well as in your professional practice. It is through good communication that professionals who work with people, be they children, young people, adults, patients or service users or other professionals, demonstrate respect, integrity, competence and an essential value base. We will now focus on the two types of interpersonal communication that inform the key concepts for this chapter.

Non-verbal communication

Because we are social beings we are nearly always on show. Being on show means that we are susceptible to other people's interpretation of our behaviours. Non-verbally, we communicate through facial expressions, hand gestures and through our physical posture, or body language. These expressions or behaviours lend themselves to others' interpretation whereby meaning is attached to behaviour. Of course, it is not only that other people interpret our behaviour but we go through the same process of ascribing meaning to other people's non-verbal behaviour. Lishman (1994, p15) draws attention to the importance of symbolic communication, that is, *behaviour, actions or communications which represent or denote something else*. These include the clothes we wear and our general appearance and the environment in which we work with people.

ACTIVITY 2.2

Thinking about and exploring the relevance of symbolic communication, consider these questions.

- What do you think the way you dress says about you? How might other people interpret or feel about the way you dress?
- Thinking about a private space like a room, what image might the room convey? Is it welcoming? Clean? Tidy?
- What about issues such as punctuality or reliability? What message might be conveyed if you are late or you don't do what you said you would?

Symbolic communication has meaning and:

represent[s] powerful aspects of our communication. They convey messages about class, culture, ethnicity and gender, power, control and authority, and about genuineness, concern, respect and caring.

(Lishman, 1994, p23)

ACTIVITY 2.3

Think back to Activity 2.1, which involved observing the behaviour of five different people.

- How did you interpret their facial expressions and gestures or behaviour?
- Justify your interpretation.

For example, if a friend is reading, how do you interpret his facial expression? Does he look as though he is concentrating? What makes you think that? Is he smiling? What emotion does that convey to you?

If you are concentrating on someone's body posture, how do you interpret that person's stance?

Koprowska (2005, p40), when citing Damasio (1999), reminds us that much non-verbal communication is learnt and culturally specific, but yet there are some emotions, known as 'universal emotions', *that all human beings experience and express . . . in the same way. They are happiness, sadness, fear, anger, surprise, and disgust, and each has a particular expression.* Equally, 'background emotions' are always present and these shape our body language, such as posture and body movement, as well as levels of animation expressed in our face.

So, in observing others' facial expression and body movements, we may feel quite confident that we have interpreted their emotions correctly. For instance, a smile might convey a sense of pleasure or happiness. Using another example, someone standing but moving from one foot to the other may indicate impatience or irritation. However, it becomes easier to interpret someone's behaviour or facial expression if we are aware of the context in which that behaviour takes place and if we are sensitive to the social and cultural context in which we are trying to make sense of that behaviour.

What we should be aware of is that, without clarifying what these behaviours mean to the person we are observing, we are making assumptions about what we think the person's behaviour means. In other words, we assume that a smiling face indicates that someone is happy, when in fact, the smile may be an attempt to mask irritation or sadness; equally, the person moving from one foot to another may be anxious rather than annoyed.

It is particularly important in developing our professional competence that we take care not to make assumptions about the person we are dealing with. Burnard (1997, p87) uses the term 'zone of fantasy' and alerts us to the danger of falling into this zone. Instead, we need to be careful about making assumptions about other people's feelings without first checking out with them that our interpretation is correct. Seeking clarity of meaning and checking our assumptions are most likely to involve the use of verbal communication skills, which will be covered later in this chapter.

Developing self-awareness of non-verbal communication for study and work

In everyday life, we can see that our non-verbal behaviours and those of others are open to interpretation and form the basis for making assumptions about others and ourselves. Indeed, this forms the basis for much of everyday life – we have learnt the process of reading other people's behaviour through socialisation and appreciating the social and cultural norms associated with facial expressions and behaviour. However, in our studies and professional lives, we need to develop sensitivity to these expressions and behaviours in such a way that we respond appropriately to others. We also want our behaviours and expressions to be understood by those who are observing or assessing us and those with whom we are working. We need to be aware of our non-verbal behaviours and behave in ways that do not lend themselves to misinterpretation. In developing our skills and professional competence, whether as a social worker, teacher or health care worker, we are talking about the presentation of the 'social' self, that is, *that aspect of the person which is shared with others.* For it is *the social self* that *is closely linked to the self-as-defined-by-others* (Burnard, 1997, p57). Non-verbal behaviours are a significant aspect by which others judge us and, in our professional roles, this is most significant for those we are seeking to assist.

Burnard (1997, p68) defines self-awareness as *the gradual and continuous process of noticing and exploring aspects of the self, whether behavioural, psychological or physical, with the intention of developing personal and interpersonal understanding.* He goes on to argue that, by becoming more self-aware, through developing a deeper understanding of ourselves, we become more sensitive of other people's experiences. This is why, at the root of developing our understanding of the range of communication skills used in professional practice, the maxim 'practise, practise, practise' is often repeatedly emphasised. It is not just that we should have a theoretical understanding of communication skills, but we also need to develop, practise and refine these skills in order to develop a range of communication skills that enable us to engage and work effectively with different service users.

Recognising non-verbal behaviours

ACTIVITY 2.4

Three people are required to complete this activity: an observer, an interviewer and someone who is prepared to be interviewed, the interviewee.

- For two minutes the interviewee has to talk about a non-sensitive subject such as the journey to university or a pleasant event.
- The interviewer is given an example of non-verbal behaviour, such as twiddling the hair, avoiding eye contact with the interviewee or persistent nodding, and is asked to act this out throughout the interview.
- The observer is asked to identify the non-verbal behaviour of the interviewer, write it down and notice if the interviewee seems to react to the interviewer's behaviour. The observer must not say anything until the interview has finished.

At the end of the interview, discuss how it felt.

- Did the interviewee notice the non-verbal behaviour? What impact did it have?
- How did the interviewer feel acting out this behaviour?
- What did the observer notice about the interview?

In some instances, non-verbal behaviour can be useful. For instance, head nodding can be an encouraging sign, indicating a 'say more' response. However, it can also be distracting, as the interviewee may feel they have said enough but are encouraged to say more to please the worker.

ACTIVITY 2.5

Ask a few friends, classmates or members of your family to observe you presenting on a topic of your choice for at least two minutes. Choose something with which you are very familiar so that you don't have to research the topic. Those observing should be prepared to give feedback on your facial expressions, mannerisms and gestures, eye contact and posture – that is, they are focusing on your non-verbal communication habits. Alternatively you can record yourself using a suitable camera or use a mirror.

Key questions for you to consider are:

- what are your non-verbal strengths?
- what areas do you need to work on?

To begin with, you may feel self-conscious about your behaviour and expressions as you practise your non-verbal communication skills, but the act of practising and constructive feedback (whether through observation or digital recording) is designed to help you enhance these skills and to achieve good outcomes. Developing self-awareness about your non-verbal communication skills will have a positive impact on your studies and is key to your successful practice.

Verbal skills

We now turn to verbal communication skills as part of the repertoire of communication skills needed in your professional role. Good verbal skills are not just about the way you speak but also include having a good vocabulary and the efficient use of language.

Once again there are numerous contexts for the use of verbal skills: presentations, meetings or seminars and a range of people with whom you may have contact through your studies or working day:

- pupil;
- parent;
- tutor;
- peers;
- nurse;
- doctor;
- ward manager;
- head of a residential home;
- patient;
- social worker;
- carer/relative;
- service user.

With some of these people, you may feel quite confident, whereas others may make you feel intimidated, which may affect the quality of your interaction with them. However, given the range of different people, it is likely that you will adapt your interpersonal skills according to their age and status, their own use of language and how they present to you, as well as adapting your style according to the purpose of your contact with them and the context in which you find yourself. All these factors are likely to influence your response.

How we verbally interact with people is also shaped by the purpose of our contact and the context in which we find ourselves. For instance, if you have to present to the whole class you may feel more aware of the fact that other people may be watching compared to presenting to just one person. The environment can also have an impact: talking in a public place may generate more anxiety than talking in a more private place.

Whatever the purpose or context of your contact with people, your verbal communication skills need to be:

- clear;
- simple;
- structured.

Clarity

In being clear you will express yourself freely, purposefully and efficiently. This requires some planning and preparation since you need to be explicit about the purpose of your contact with that person and to communicate your purpose to that individual. In your studies and professional role you should avoid ambiguities about why you are involved or a lack of clarity as to why you need the information you are asking for. For example, when going for a tutorial with a tutor you should be clear not only about what you want to discuss but also how you are going to express this. You need to understand your needs, what the tutor can offer, what a tutorial is and how to articulate or express this.

Simplicity

Being simple is not about being patronising towards people with whom we are involved, but it does require us to think about our use of language, avoid jargon and speak to people in ways that are age-appropriate and appropriate to that person's developmental ability. So in working with children or young people or people with learning difficulties or mental impairments, we should talk to them in ways which match their ability to understand what we are saying. Equally, with people whose first language is not English or those who have a sensory impairment, we will need to think about alternative forms of communication that are appropriate for their needs, such as a professional interpreter or signer, in order to avoid disadvantaging people who require these services. With your tutor you will use language appropriate to your studies and analytical abilities. In all verbal contact with people you are aiming for mutual understanding.

Structure

Structure is achieved through planning and preparation since knowing what you need to say and how you are going to say it helps to form a plan of approach. Think about this chapter and book more generally. If we discussed non-verbal communication and then moved on to a completely unrelated topic, such as society, before returning to verbal communication, then the impact of the message would be lessened and the meaning lost. Good structure reduces the possibility of confusion and enhances the likelihood of good outcomes.

Expanding your vocabulary

As alluded to above, in being clear, simple and structured it is essential to use the correct language for the person and context. The importance of lexicon, or a good vocabulary, is emphasised because it is through the judicious use of words and language that we are certain of clarity and that our role, purpose and meaning are understood. Consider, for example, the use of the word 'judicious' in the previous sentence. Of course, another word could have been used to convey a similar meaning – perhaps 'prudent' or 'considerate' or 'thoughtful' or 'discerning'. However, 'judicious' conveys the meaning of all of these and more, including that we use judgment in our choice of words and language. One word is used to convey several concepts about the use of words and language simply and with clarity.

There are a number of ways to expand your lexicon, including through the development of your reading skills and listening – in particular, the notion of active listening.

Reading does many things: it is used as escapism, to introduce us to different cultures and to enhance our knowledge. The more widely you read, the more likely you are to encounter words that are outside your everyday use. It is beneficial to read a range of texts that you would not normally engage with, perhaps a quality newspaper, poetry or a different genre of novel. There are also many digital means of doing this, including downloads of full texts. The overall aim in reading more widely is to engage with words, language and texts and to develop your vocabulary for your studies and later work.

Another method of enhancing lexicon is to listen, both to yourself and to others. If you record how you speak or read out loud something that you have written you will be able to listen later and hear the patterns and nuances in your language, for example, if you frequently use a favourite word or use colloquialisms. Listening to unfamiliar radio programmes can also be helpful and there are many programmes, not just news programmes, that deal with social and political issues in which current and sometimes controversial topics are debated articulately. There is a great deal of content on channels such as BBC Radio 4 that considers issues such as morals and ethics, disability, law and policy and education. Many others include use of language, for example in discussions of literature, embracing fiction and poetry. Once again these may be available digitally through downloads such as podcasts.

Wider reading, listening actively to yourself and to such programmes is a key step in developing lexicon. The following activities will help you think about this further.

ACTIVITY 2.6

Thinking about your reading preferences, undertake the following activities.

- Write down the most common type of newspaper, magazine and book that you read. What do you read most often and why?
- Read a number of online articles and reports from a quality newspaper or news agency that are appropriate to your studies. Write down any new or unfamiliar words and look up their meaning.
- Look up the current top-selling fiction and non-fiction titles (accessible online or in some Sunday newspapers). Identify a book or an author you would not usually read and buy or borrow a book and read it.

ACTIVITY 2.7

In order to explore your use of language, read out loud to yourself something that you have written. Write down what you notice about your use of language and words, using the following prompt questions:

- What does your writing sound like?
- Does what you heard reflect what you wanted to say?
- Do you use a word or phrase commonly?

- Is your writing clear, simple and structured?
- What different words might you have used?

Now read the same piece to one or more other people and ask them for feedback, using the same questions on your use of language and words. What have you learned?

ACTIVITY 2.8

In order to develop your lexicon through listening, listen to a radio programme that you would not normally listen to but not one that is focused on music. Many of these programmes are available via the internet using playback functions so even late-night programmes can be listened to at a more convenient time.

Listen to the words used by the presenters and correspondents and make a note of unfamiliar terms. Look these words up in a dictionary and consider if they might be useful for your studies and practice.

Dictionaries and other tools

Developing your skills as a student and a practitioner involves listening with a purpose; not only will you be attempting to determine meaning and what is being defined and to interpret and develop questions, but you will also be expanding your vocabulary and use of words. Two crucial outcomes of an appropriate lexicon are an enhanced ability to put other people's work into your own words within your assessed academic work and the potential for better outcomes for those in need of your assistance. Where you can explain with clarity your role and purpose you are more likely to develop effective partnerships with clients, service users, patients and colleagues and professionals from other agencies and settings. You are also likely to be better understood when arguing for a particular course of action or for scarce resources.

As the exercises above suggest, an improved lexicon is not something that will develop by osmosis, that is by some sort of magical assimilation of new words and phrases – you will need to develop this actively. A good dictionary and thesaurus will be invaluable in understanding the meaning and use of unfamiliar or technical words. These are available either in book form or in online versions but take care that whatever you use is appropriate to your context, for example UK English and not US English, or vice versa. You will also have the choice of a general dictionary and a specialist dictionary and there are many arguments for having access to both, particularly as a general dictionary is unlikely to include some of the specialist terms used in the social sciences or professions allied to medicine.

It is also a good idea to write new words down (as suggested in the activities above) and to develop your own resources. Concept cards or index cards, whether in paper or electronic form, can be used to record a new word, its definition and its appropriate use, for example:

Osmosis

Definition: The unconscious process of acquiring something, such as ideas or knowledge, by absorption or assimilation.

Use: He never reads a book or studies but gets good marks; he must learn by osmosis.

Alternatives: A technical term in the physical sciences describing the absorption of a solvent through a membrane from a less concentrated solution to a higher concentrated solution so that the solution on either side of the membrane is of the same concentration.

ACTIVITY 2.9

To begin the development of a word resource, consider the term 'colloquialisms' used above and complete a concept card entry using the suggested headings:

- Definition:
- Use:
- Alternatives:

Active listening and good communication

So far, in thinking about verbal communication skills, that is, our use of words or language, we have emphasised the need for clear and simple communication and a good lexicon so that the other person understands what is said, minimising opportunities for misinterpretation. We have also highlighted the need to structure what you communicate in a way that aids understanding and clarity. The person you are talking to needs to follow what is being said and it needs to be presented in such a way that it makes sense to that person.

Additionally, the need for clarity and structure in our verbal communication means we need to be aware of the impact of what we say and how we present ourselves. This calls to mind the importance of remembering our body language, including facial and body gestures and how these are used to convey that you are listening, as well as the use of those features of communication known as 'paralinguistics'. This is defined as those aspects of speech that are not words and includes:

- quality of voice;
- volume;
- intonation and pitch;
- rate of speech;
- tone of voice;
- conversational oil – that is, utterances such as 'uh-huh', 'mm-hmm', 'I see' (Williams, 1997, pp17–20).

Effective communication requires not just listening but active listening skills in order to develop the lexicon essential for good outcomes, make sense of what is going on (is a person's body language in tune with what is being said?) and to acknowledge that communication is a two-way process. Just as you draw upon your knowledge and understanding of both verbal and non-verbal communication skills to listen actively to what is said and to interpret whether body language matches the verbalised sentiments, so does the other person engaged in the dialogue. Thompson (2009, p105) suggests active listening involves:

- acknowledging feelings;
- appropriate use of body language;

- resisting the temptation to interrupt;
- paying careful attention to what is being said in order to avoid misunderstanding;
- avoiding jumping to conclusion or relying on stereotypes;
- reflecting back key points of what has been said to confirm understanding.

REFLECTION POINT

In your role as the interviewer, use Activity 2.4 to consider more specifically and reflect upon the use of explicit active listening skills. This time avoid the exaggerated behaviour you were asked to display.

Reflecting on your performance, consider the following questions:

- How do you convey your understanding of the situation to the person you are interviewing?
- What facial expressions might denote interest, understanding or sympathy?
- How do you oil the flow of conversation when you are listening? Is this helpful or distracting?
- Do you tend to nod or smile?
- How do you seat yourself when engaged in an interview?
- What signals might your body posture convey? Are you comfortable, relaxed or tense?
- Do you gesticulate? What impact might this have on the person you are listening to?
- What emotion does the tone of your voice convey? Do you sound sympathetic, patronising, bored, shocked?
- Do you speak clearly or adopt a particular tone when you talk to different people?
- How do you hide your shock or embarrassment when someone tells you something that has that kind of impact on you?

Such considerations form part of your learning and the development of self-awareness about communication skills. Active listening is complex and demanding – you have to learn the subtleties of how your verbal and non-verbal communications can be interpreted as well as being aware of the impact of symbolic communications and present yourself in ways that are conducive to context and the purpose of your interactions with people. Equally, however, your own verbal and non-verbal communication skills are being interpreted by the people you are working with: just as you have to listen, observe and interpret people's behaviour and responses, they in turn go through the same process of trying to make sense of you and forming a judgment about your capabilities and the profession you represent.

This is why communication skills are so central to your role – you cannot practise professionally unless you communicate effectively. As a result, communication skills are a central part of your learning within your programme of study and it is essential to practise and develop them. Of course this should all take place within what Hanley (2009, p188) identifies as *safe learning environments*; Hanley suggests that classroom environments are appropriate for learning communication skills if your tutor takes care to create an environment that is safe, with clear expectations about behaviour and learning aims in order to encourage participative and informative learning. This allows for a setting in which communication skills can be practised and nurtured without harming oneself or others. Together these factors allow for learning to be facilitated through practice and the development of a repertoire of communication skills and different styles of approach that enable you to work with different people with different needs.

Alternative communication approaches

Not all people speak and not all body language is commonly used or understood throughout the world. Whilst the majority of cultures are concerned with appearance and dress because these convey messages about attraction, modesty and status, the use and interpretation of movement, posture and facial expressions can differ greatly. Eye contact illustrates this effectively: Western cultures tend to view eye contact positively and can feel snubbed or that the conversational partner lacks interest if there is no or too little eye contact. However in Japan and parts of Africa and Latin America, eye contact may be avoided as a sign of respect. Conversely, some Arabic cultures will maintain prolonged eye contact as a demonstration of interest and understanding of what is being communicated but this may make those from Western cultures uneasy, interpreting it as too attentive and perhaps an indication of sexual interest. It is easy to appreciate the importance of understanding the cultural context to avoid embarrassment and offence.

It is also important to point out that not all languages are verbal and for many people signs are used as the primary form of communication. This may be through formal languages such as British Sign Language (BSL) or American Sign Language or through augmentative or alternative systems such as Makaton, Blissymbolics, Rebus, Picture Communication Symbols (PCS) and image vocabulary. Written communication can also take the form of characters that are not the recognisable letters of the Roman alphabet, for example Braille and the Moon alphabet. Sign languages are as varied as spoken language and it is quite common to encounter regional as well as international variations. For example, deaf people in the north of Ireland may use Irish Sign Language in preference to BSL.

It is not possible within this chapter to consider the range of sign languages or available augmentative or alternative systems but you should spend a little time making yourself familiar with these and their constituency and purpose.

ACTIVITY 2.10
Explore the internet for the items listed below in order to research and consider augmentative and alternative communication systems:

- BSL;
- Braille and Moon;
- Makaton;
- Blissymbolics;
- Rebus;
- PCS;
- Image vocabulary.

In particular, note:

- Why were they developed and who are the intended users of each language or system?
- What complexities are involved with each? What caution should you be aware of?
- Where can you find out more?

CHAPTER SUMMARY

- Verbal and non-verbal communication skills together with the importance of active listening skills are emphasised as a complex and active process of engagement alongside developing your lexicon.
- These skills need to be practised and developed so that you become skilled in their use and interpretation and use them in ways that allow people to engage with you with trust and confidence.
- You should also remember that body language is not homogenous and certain gestures and expressions may have different emphasis and meanings for different cultures.
- You should be aware of alternative languages and augmentative communication systems and that these too can vary by region and nation and may have been designed for particular groups of users.
- The activities in this chapter are designed to help you make links between your learning and practice development.

The following two chapters continue the theme of communication, with Chapter 3 concentrating on developing information literacy, thinking, reading and writing skills.

FURTHER READING

Koprowska, J (2005) *Communication and Interpersonal Skills in Social Work*. Exeter: Learning Matters.

Thompson, N (2009) *People Skills* (3rd edition). Basingstoke: Palgrave.

Williams, D (1997) *Communications Skills in Practice: A practical guide for health professionals*. London: Jessica Kingsley.

These books are useful introductory texts that focus on developing your understanding of why such skills are important in the helping professions and provide useful practical exercises to engage in.

3 INFORMATION LITERACY, THINKING, READING AND WRITING

CHAPTER OBJECTIVES

By the end of this chapter you should be able to:

- know how to access the literature and information that you need for your studies;

- reflect upon your experiences of using information and communication technology (ICT) for your studies;

- develop your thinking skills to achieve a successful assessment outcome;

- draw upon strategies to enhance reading and writing skills for your studies and future practice.

Introduction

This chapter covers four key skills necessary for successful study. Learning involves analysing and evaluating existing information and developing a critique or argument that produces new information. In part one of this chapter we consider how to use ICT to find relevant books and articles and the thinking skills required to consider the relevance and validity of this literature. Part two leads on to consider skills for reading and writing and, with particular focus on essay writing, aims to help you produce work that meets the various requirements of an assessment.

It might seem obvious to state that the ability to use technology and thinking are core skills for a successful student; however, to do these in an academically appropriate way requires consideration and practice. Search the internet using a generic search engine and you are likely to come up with thousands of useless references but to undertake a search that is specific and relevant to the topic you are researching requires understanding of what the relevant information might be and how your tutors expect you to use the information you find. This will be articulated through module learning and assessment outcomes, typically expressed using terms such as 'critically analyse', 'evaluate' or 'synthesise', which clearly indicate the need to think about what you have learned and to compare and contrast the ideas explored in your work for assessment.

Germane to the ability to use technology and to think about the information found is the ability to understand your personal thoughts and feelings about the task you are undertaking. Emotional intelligence refers to your aptitude in being aware of your feelings and the feelings of others, for motivating yourself on the basis of this understanding and for managing your emotions for your benefit and that of others (Goleman, 1998, p317). Whilst there are aspects of emotional intelligence that are contested, it is accepted that your experience of your studies and work with people is fundamentally emotional. We are certain that you will be able to recall times during your education when there were incidents evoking either, for example, a heightened sense of well-being or anxiety. Certainly working with vulnerable people and those in need requires the ability to communicate, not only verbally but also with empathy and in recognition of their emotional state. We urge you throughout your use of this book and in your studies not only to refer to the approaches to study and practice discussed here but also to remain vigilant about the impact of emotions.

In part two of this chapter we will consider reading and writing skills and suggest activities to enhance your awareness of your attitude and approach to each. However, before you read or write anything you need to ensure that you are using appropriate and relevant material; inevitably you will use university information technology systems and processes as well as the internet to find what you need. Information literacy recognises both the skill in using the technology and your ability to reflect upon your experience, your thoughts and feelings to discern the different ways in which you approach the use of ICT.

It is important to remember that study need not be a solitary activity and tutors are available to offer advice and guidance to help you achieve your aims in undertaking your studies. Sometimes this advice is also offered by specialist study skills tutors within a school or faculty or by a central skills unit within the college or university. If you do not wish to speak to a tutor most universities will publish, both in paper form and online, information sheets on topics such as using the library and undertaking electronic searches. You are strongly advised to make yourself familiar with, and if necessary to make use of, these resources.

PART ONE

Information literacy

Whatever your course or your intended profession, you will need to find information from an increasingly diverse range of sources, often through electronic methods, and to discern what is useful and what is not. Communication skills and information technology skills operate in parallel and are necessary attributes of the successful student and practitioner. The former recognises your ability to perform more widely as a competent student, as discussed in Chapter 2. The latter focuses more specifically on information literacy; that is, your relationship with ICT, your ability to recognise why information is needed, what information is needed, how to access this information and how to evaluate it. As a competent student you are expected to plan and reflect upon what influences the quality of your search performance (Bruce et al., 2006, p7). You also need to know how to use libraries and electronic resources, including how information is stored, managed and retrieved and furthermore to think about the information accessed and how to analyse, evaluate and synthesise it.

Bruce et al. (p6) cite research by Edwards and Bruce (2006) that identifies a relational model of four categories that capture students' different ways of searching and learning to search for internet information. These are:

- *Information searching is seen as looking for a needle in a haystack.*
- *Information searching is seen as finding a way through a maze.*
- *Information searching is seen as using the tools as a filter.*
- *Information searching is seen as panning for gold.*

Edwards and Bruce conclude that students possess and experience all four categories, but the use of a specific one, at a particular time, is determined by the context of the search. Categories three and four are positively oriented and hint at success, direction and momentum in the search whereas categories one and two engender a sense of frustration, perhaps of futility, and certainly an awareness of the potential to lose your way. Whilst it is desirable to work within categories three and four, this will not always be your experience, perhaps because you are unfamiliar with the technology or processes or are uncertain of the specific requirements and objectives of the search. Information-literate students who identify that they are working in category one or two will want to enhance their experience in order to achieve category three or four. In these circumstances it is necessary to reflect upon your approach to the search and, where necessary, to undertake activities that enhance your awareness, understanding and capabilities. It is possible to discern similarities between the qualities expected of the information-literate student and emotional intelligence, specifically in relation to ICT; that is, the ability to recognise your thoughts and emotions in using the technology; the impact that these have on you and others (for example, if you are part of a group) and how you deal with this knowledge – ultimately how you learn.

REFLECTION POINT

Thinking about your own experience of searching for internet information for academic purposes, in which of the four categories identified above would you place yourself?

Comment

It is important to acknowledge the importance of reflection to the concepts of information literacy and emotional intelligence. Students utilising categories one or two need to reflect on their experience if they wish to develop their information search into a category three or four outcome. Reflection is dealt with in more detail in Chapter 6 but engaging with the reflective activities throughout the book will help to enhance your understanding of your information literacy and emotional intelligence.

The Society of College, National and University Libraries (SCONUL, 1999, p8) has produced a set of seven 'headline' skills that help to define information literacy. These are combined in Table 3.1 with other skills models to show diagrammatically the relationships between someone who is able to use ICT competently and the reflective process. The 'pillars' of the SCONUL model represent an iterative process (where each stage builds upon the previous one) so that students progress through competency from baseline to expertise by practising the skills and reflecting upon this experience.

LUPTON'S STUDENTS' WAYS OF EXPERIENCING INFORMATION LITERACY	MOON'S REFLECTION IN LEARNING	MAYER–SALOVEY FOUR-BRANCH MODEL OF EMOTIONAL INTELLIGENCE	SCONUL HEADLINE SKILLS FOR INFORMATION LITERACY
Category 3 – Learning as a social responsibility Information literacy is experienced when researching an essay as *applying learning to help solve individual or societal problems.* Subcategories: (a) Helping the community (b) Effecting social and political change	**Transformative learning** There is recognition that the personal frame of reference can change according to one's emotional state. The views and motives of others are taken into account and compared against the self. There is a deliberate internal dialogue	**Reflective regulation of emotions to promote emotional and intellectual growth** Ability to engage emotions reflectively in relation to oneself and others. Emotions prioritise thinking by directing attention to important information	7. The ability to synthesise and build upon existing information, contributing to the creation of new knowledge
Category 2 – Developing an argument Information literacy is experienced when researching an essay as *using background information to develop an argument* Subcategories:	**Meaning-making** There is description of the activity but external ideas are considered and there is evidence of analysis. The worth of exploring motives is accepted and there is an ability to be critical of action	**Understanding and analysing emotions; employing emotional knowledge** Ability to label emotions and to interpret the meanings that emotions convey	6. The ability to organise, apply and communicate information to others in ways appropriate to the situation 5. The ability to compare and evaluate information obtained from different sources

Lupton (2004)	Moon (1999)	Mayer and Salovey (1997)	SCONUL (1999)
(a) Learning about the topic (b) Setting the topic in a context (c) Rethinking the argument		**Emotional facilitation of thinking** Emotional states differentially encourage specific problem-solving approaches	4. The ability to locate and access information
Category 1 – Seeking evidence Information literacy is experienced when researching an essay as *seeking evidence to back up an existing argument.* Subcategory: (c) Seeking contrasting perspectives	**Making sense** Coherence is sought and attention begins to be paid to one's own feelings and the views of others		3. The ability to construct strategies for locating information 2. The ability to distinguish ways in which the information 'gap' may be addressed 1. The ability to recognise a need for information
Category 1 – Seeking evidence Information literacy is experienced when researching an essay as *seeking evidence to back up an existing argument.* Subcategories: (a) Seeking statistics (b) Seeking opinions and ideas	**Noticing** Characterised by a descriptive account and little reflection. Some mention of emotional reactions but no consideration of emotions on behaviour. One activity considered at a time but ideas are not linked, nor are external influences considered	**Perception, appraisal and expression of emotion** Ability to identify emotion in one's physical states, feelings and thoughts	

Table 3.1 **Comparison of Lupton (2004), Moon (1999), Mayer and Salovey (1997) and SCONUL (1999) skills models**

SCONUL, Society of College, National and University Libraries.

Finding information and literature

The internet and advances in ICT mean that there is more information available than you can usefully utilise or make sense of. Many of you will be operating at the lower levels described in Table 3.1 and may be confused about how to use new search tools such as databases effectively. You need to develop effective search strategies and to be discerning in your approach and choice of relevant material. Discussions with tutors about the task they have set will help with this initially and will work towards realisation of the first of the SCONUL skills. Tutors will be particularly interested in you accessing and reading relevant books and academic journals. Activity 3.1 will help you to begin to appreciate skill two: the ability to distinguish ways in which the information 'gap' may be addressed.

ACTIVITY 3.1

Your tutor has asked you to develop an essay plan on the topic of safeguarding vulnerable children or adults. Part of your task is to write down the potential sources of information for your essay.

- Start by listing the types of information you might need before considering where you can find this information.
- Divide the sources into web-based and non-web-based sources.

Comment

Your approach to this activity is likely to begin with an appraisal of your own knowledge of the topic and the various gateways to information, however it is a good idea for even a confident researcher to write down and thus make explicit what you think you know. In this way you can begin to check assumptions and identify any gaps in your knowledge. A typical result for this task is demonstrated in Table 3.2, although this is an illustration and you may have thought of additional types of information and sources.

Some of the sources for the information you require are likely to be already familiar – books, websites, newspapers – but others less so, including databases and subject gateways. A database is simply a large store of records for information that might be useful to you, including journal abstracts; it requires you to use relevant search terms to access this information. A subject gateway is a web-based resource that enables you to search the internet focused on a particular specialism. It will reference a wide range of sources of information, including books, journals and websites.

ACTIVITY 3.2

Take a look at the following examples of a database and subject gateway. What do you notice about how these resources work?

- database: www.apa.org/psycinfo/;
- subject gateway: www.intute.ac.uk.

INFORMATION REQUIRED	NON-WEB-BASED SOURCES	WEB-BASED SOURCES
Contemporary/current issues	Tutor and other academics/ researchers at university Journal articles Newspapers and magazines	Databases/subject gateways ejournals Government websites Local and international agency websites, e.g. NSPCC, EU, UN
Historical perspectives	Library – books Subject librarian Theses	Electronic books Agency websites, e.g. NSPCC
Theories and models of intervention	Library – books Subject librarian Tutor and other academics	Electronic books Databases ejournals
Policies and procedures	Government publications Local agency guidelines	Government websites Agency websites, e.g. Local Safeguarding Children Board
Law	Government publications Books	Government and local and international agency websites Legal websites, e.g. Children's Legal Centre
Statistics	Government and agency publications	Government and local and international agency websites
User/client perspectives	Newspapers Books Agency publications	Agency websites ejournals Databases
International perspectives	Books Conferences International agency publications	International agency websites Conference proceedings ejournals

Table 3.2 **Types of information and their sources for Activity 3.1**

NSPCC, National Society for Prevention of Cruelty to Children; EU, European Union; UN, United Nations.

Comment

You are unlikely to be able to search using the database listed in Activity 3.2 as you require permission or a membership to do so. Access is granted to you free of charge by your university or college who pay a fee on your behalf. It is also useful to bear in mind that access to databases is straightforward when using computers on campus but when you are working off campus you may need to accept a 'cookie' (a simple text file sent to your computer) from your university that recognises you as a student. In addition you may need to access the database through an additional link such as Athens or Shibboleth. Don't worry about these just now as your university library will provide full information, but do remember to ask.

Having decided on the nature of the information you require and where to find it, you will embark on a search. However, caution is required before embarking on your electronic hunt as it is necessary to understand the rigour that is required at university level of your ability not only to find information but also to appraise it, including questioning the relevance of the information, and subsequently to use it appropriately. You need to develop a search strategy that involves successful and logical navigation of a number of sources, followed by applied decision-making aimed at filtering out superfluous information from that which is relevant before pulling the information together from the various sources and developing a coherent argument. Achieving this level of rigour in your approach to ICT is evidence that your work is valid, reliable, accurate and credible.

At university you can seek the advice of your tutor or of a subject librarian. However, there will be many times when you are working alone on the internet and have to make decisions about the appropriateness of your search strategy and the quality of the information you access. It pays to remember a few things about the internet.

- Anybody from anywhere in the world can upload information.
- This information may be inaccurate or anecdotal.
- It can also be changed, manipulated or removed very easily.

Using keywords

Use of the internet can provide a challenge in meeting the academic demands made of you and your work. A good way to overcome some of these pitfalls at the outset is to think of some of the keywords relevant to the task set.

In Activity 3.1 you were asked to plan an essay on the topic of safeguarding vulnerable children or adults. If you were to focus on children your keywords would include 'safeguarding', 'vulnerable' and 'children'. However using these broad terms is likely to lead to many potential sources of information which you will need to reduce to a manageable and relevant number. You should also think of other words that are specific to your focus, for example, if researching law and policy, your search terms might be 'safeguarding', 'children', 'policy', 'law' and 'UK' – the latter particularly relevant to limiting the geographical range of the search. If you were in particular considering children under five you might substitute the word 'children' with the term 'early years'. You might also want to limit your search to a particular period of time, for example '2000 to 2012'. The point is that you should try to be as specific as possible to enhance the relevance of your search returns.

Keywords are used by libraries in the cataloguing of books and by journals in sorting articles. They are a key component of a search strategy and many search engines, particularly those of databases, use them. You will also be offered the opportunity to undertake a basic search or an advanced search: the latter allows you to use more keywords and to be more specific with your search criteria. However you also need to be careful that you do not exclude what might be relevant information from your results because of the words you use. For example, use of the keyword 'children' could, depending on the search engine, exclude information that uses the term 'child'. An advanced search will offer the opportunity to use Boolean operators. The first of these is AND, so you can search for 'children' AND 'safeguarding', meaning that both of these terms must be present in the records found. The second of the terms is OR: this allows you to search for 'child' OR 'children' with either term being present in the records found. The third term is NOT: a search using 'children' NOT 'adults' will result in records that do not include the word adults. An asterix (*) is also a useful search tool because the term 'child*' means that all words with the root 'child' will be identified and the search will return records that include the words 'child', 'child's', 'children' and 'children's'. Finally, in using keywords you should be mindful of spelling and which forms of English are being used, for example, behaviour (UK spelling)/behavior (US spelling). Different terms may also be used in different countries or jurisdictions.

Thinking about the literature

Your decision about the usefulness of the information will depend on a number of factors, including your ability to analyse it and your level of study.

Analysis necessarily involves consideration of several questions to test the quality of the information, including: is it relevant to your aims? Do any biases exist? Were the data gathered in an appropriate way? Who gathered the information and did they use reliable sources?

You will only find information relevant if it is suitable to your aims and this includes making sure that data cover the area you are interested in in terms of both geography and focus. There is no point, for example, in seeking information on safeguarding children in a UK context by looking at research from France or Germany, unless the task set requires you to do this. There is also little point in using data on safeguarding children if your focus is on safeguarding adults. A final consideration in relation to relevance concerns the level of the information. Textbooks and articles are written for many different audiences and by authors with different levels of knowledge and expertise. A secondary school text on health and social care is unlikely to cover the topic you are researching in sufficient depth if you are writing a dissertation in your final year.

In addition to considering the authors' knowledge and level of expertise it is also reasonable to question whether or not there are any biases in their work. Biases can occur for example because the work is funded in a particular way or by a particular agency, including the government. An illustration of this is the controversy over the UK government's use of research into drug use and the danger of drugs during the winter of 2009 that led to the resignation of several scientist advisers. The personal, political and moral views of the authors may also influence the data. Those opposed to euthanasia may emphasise research that supports their view of the world whereas those who support the right to choose the manner of our death are likely to use data that support their view. It is also important to acknowledge that your own views, morals and prejudices can influence your choice of information and you should reflect upon this as you are undertaking your search.

There is a need also to question the nature of the method used to collect the data. Researchers who prefer to use more scientific methods in their approach to the question of safeguarding children or adults would include consideration of prevalence and utilise facts and figures from a range of sources. On the other hand, researchers who favour an approach that takes account of both the thoughts and feelings of the children and adults involved (and also of the researchers themselves) would shy away from such a quantitative approach. These are very different ways of considering the same phenomenon and there is no right or wrong. However there may be arguments about the validity of the method used and your own views and professional context may favour one over the other – broadly, although not exclusively, the first approach is seen most commonly in medicine whilst, in the social sciences, the second approach is typical.

Questions can subsequently be asked of the authors' sample size and subsequent claims. Is it appropriate for an author to claim that a finding applies to all vulnerable older people if the sample consisted of only six women aged 60–65? What about older women or women from different cultural, religious or social backgrounds? What about older men? In this example you are asking if the sample is representative of the population in general. Related to this are questions of how the sample was chosen and the method used, including what questions were asked. Consider the following questions:

- Do you believe in freedom of speech?
- Should paedophiles be able to discuss their practices in their own newspaper?

If your answers to these questions are different, ask yourself why.

Authors may also use secondary sources of information, such as information posted on the internet, but as we have already noted, anybody can post information there without checks on reliability, accuracy or quality. Information from credible sources such as textbooks and peer-reviewed journals is thus more highly thought of than unattributable internet sources.

'Lower-order' and 'higher-order' thinking

In addition to questions over the quality of the information you should consider the level of your current skills and abilities and your level of study. As stated above, a question or task set by a tutor will include a verb or verbs that set out the tutor's requirements and expectations – for example, analyse, evaluate, synthesise, critique – and because these are made explicit to you in the form of learning outcomes, you are able to make a judgment in relation to your own abilities. The choice of verbs is drawn from a revision of Bloom's *Taxonomy of Educational Objectives* (Anderson and Krathwohl, 2001; Figure 3.1). This approach recognises that the student will move from lower-order to higher-order thinking skills.

You cannot apply information unless you first understand it and you cannot understand it unless you remember it, and so on. The latter also implies the ability to access and retrieve information. Activity 3.3 will help you to think about the implications of the taxonomy.

ACTIVITY 3.3
For each of the words listed in Figure 3.1, starting with remembering, write a list of verbs that further explain its meaning. You will find a thesaurus helpful.

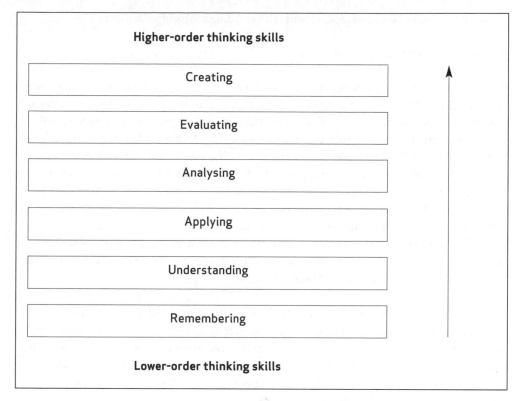

Figure 3.1 **Thinking skills**

Source: Anderson and Krathwohl (2001).

Comment

Lower-order thinking skills such as remembering and understanding will feature in some of your first assignments, whereas evaluating and creating can be expected in your final undergraduate year. Undertaking a course of study involves the development of skills over the period of your studies and you should continue to reflect upon your progress in this regard.

Remembering involves the recall of what has been learned, for example, the ability to bring to mind theories of human growth and development. Understanding involves not only remembering the theories but demonstrating your comprehension, interpretation and the meaning of the theories in your own words. Of course, as a competent student and practitioner you will be expected not only to understand but also to apply this understanding in a range of contexts in both university and practice. The ability to question the usefulness of the information and to analyse it has been discussed above and this is a necessary prerequisite to evaluating the information through critique or the development of a hypothesis. A critique or new hypothesis is indicative of the creation of new knowledge and higher-order thinking skills.

The development of thinking skills and the move from lower-order to higher-order skills requires practice, particularly if you aren't naturally curious or inquisitive. Do you, for example, read a newspaper article and find yourself disagreeing with the content, or do you watch current affairs and news-based programmes to keep up to date with issues of the day? Consider the following statement:

Reading a broadsheet newspaper is better than reading a tabloid newspaper.

Do you agree? Give reasons for your answer.

Of course, we are not simply suggesting that one type of newspaper is better than another. Any consideration of this matter and that of freedom of speech, as discussed above, requires thought but we are asking you to be explicit about your approach. Thinking about your answers to the above questions, do you think your answers are indicative of lower- or higher-order skills? You may feel confident about your answer or worry about giving the wrong answer. Context is important; you may have reached your answer to these questions very quickly but it could be that you are basing your answer on feelings, experience and common sense. Perhaps you took a little longer to think over the issues, to explore, for example, the purpose of tabloids and broadsheets, to think about their readership, the deemed value attached to the depth of the journalism or to compare the headline and the reporting of the same story in one of each type of newspaper. The latter approach suggests someone who has engaged with the question and who has taken time to consider a range of issues and views.

A starting point in developing your thinking skills is to ask if you are sufficiently engaged with the question. Have you looked for and understood alternative points of view? Have your own views been challenged or changed? Have you learned anything new or are you able to challenge perceived wisdom? Are you able to put forward your own point of view and to defend your position? You will come to appreciate that knowledge is not static; it is ever-developing and you are part of the process of this development.

As we have suggested, thinking improves with practice, just as skills in other walks of life do. It is an activity that pervades all aspects of your life, not just your studies. You can begin to develop your thinking skills by changing your habits. For example, read a newspaper or book that you would not normally be attracted to – perhaps read some poetry. This may make you initially feel awkward and uncomfortable, but recognise these feelings and think about what you need to do to overcome them. Whatever happens, do not give up easily; persistence is important. One approach might be to work with a small group of others, to read the same material and to discuss both what has been read and tactics for completing the task. In many reading groups one member will take responsibility for setting a number of questions for the group to consider.

Strategies for thinking

We have already put forward some useful ideas to help you develop your thinking skills and we think that you will also find the following strategies helpful. The six-step MASTER plan developed by Rose and Nicholl (1998) offers a step-by-step process to a question or problem. MASTER is a mnemonic for motivate, acquire, search, trigger, exhibit, reflect:

M Do you have the motivation to learn? Are you in the right frame of mind?

Preparation is important in terms of materials and resources but also in relation to attitude and understanding of the task, knowing what it is you are trying to achieve and why. Environment should also be considered: an uncomfortable chair or constant interruptions can be demotivating.

A   Acquiring the data involves information literacy, as discussed above, skills in using the technology and awareness of your thoughts and feelings when undertaking the task.

S   Searching involves working with meaning, not just learning by rote. You will be moving from a surface approach to learning to a deep approach, as discussed in Chapter 1.

T   What will your trigger be to enable you to recall from your memory what has been learned? This might involve a mnemonic, such as the one being used here, or mind maps, discussed below.

E   Exhibiting involves the explicit use of your knowledge so that the ideas and issues are being used and developed. This might include discussion with friends, family, peers or tutors. Be prepared to test your understanding.

R   Reflecting on what you have done and how you have done it is a good foundation for future learning. Chapter 6 will consider reflection in greater depth.

REFLECTION POINT

- Think back to some recent learning you have done and review your approach and experience of this learning using the six-step MASTER plan.
- Consider your weaknesses and strengths against each of the six steps.

For many of you, it can be helpful to ensure that you are using as much of your cognitive capacity as possible and this necessarily involves using that part of the brain that is logical and likes lists as well as that part of the brain that is artistic and likes diagrams. Mind maps (Buzan and Buzan, 2006) are an effective way of bringing together your logical and artistic faculties. A mind map is like a spider diagram; it allows you to move away from a linear view of a problem to a more complex view. Mind maps are intended to increase your efficiency and effectiveness.

Mind maps can be drawn by hand or there are a range of electronic mind-mapping programs, all using the same approach in the production of the map. Mind maps should begin at the centre of a page with a statement and, if possible, a drawing or picture of the topic. Thick, colourful branches (using a different colour for each branch) then grow out from the centre, each branch representing an idea that relates to the topic stated in the middle. Again, the ideas should be stated at the end of each branch and drawings or pictures used where possible. Figure 3.2 is for illustration only and we recommend that you look at other examples in books or online.

ACTIVITY 3.4

Try your own mind map. Pick your own topic or use the one from Activity 3.1 – safeguarding vulnerable children. First, use the approach that you would usually adopt if planning for an essay; after you have done this, develop a mind map. How did they compare?

Hopefully you have a range of ideas to consider when discussing the issue you chose.

Step one – Write your topic in the middle of the page and illustrate with a picture or drawing (not done here). Use colour.

UNIVERSITY

Step two – Develop a number of branches that will represent an idea related to the topic. Use illustrations and different colours for each branch.

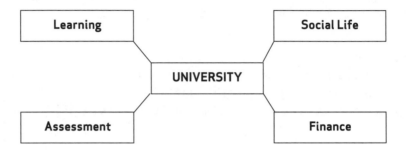

Step three – Each idea is further broken down into smaller sub-branches that represent elements of the main idea.

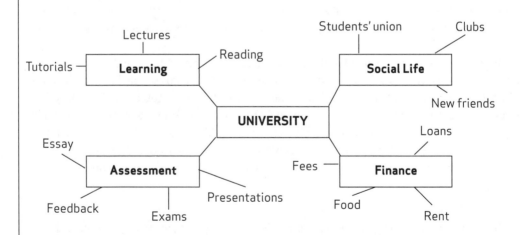

Step four – from each sub-heading developing a number of further headings as necessary

Figure 3.2 **Illustration of the development of a mind map**

PART ONE SUMMARY

- You need to develop your understanding of how you use ICT to search for relevant literature or information, adopting an applied and systematic approach.
- To limit your chances of uncovering unreliable information you should use subject gateways and databases. Being explicit about your search terms and using keywords alongside learning how to use search engines will increase your effectiveness.
- Once you have found and read the relevant information and literature, you need to understand what is required of you to produce a reliable piece of work.
- As you progress through your studies you will be expected to think about the information much more deeply but also to generate new information. The ability to question what you have read, to interrogate the authors' methodology and conclusions and to reflect upon the experience will enhance your ability to MASTER thinking.

PART TWO

In this part of the chapter we are considering reading and writing skills. Once you have found the information you require you will need to read it and write about it, commonly in the form of an essay. Active reading and good writing for university also involve thinking and the approaches discussed in part one of this chapter are relevant to the development of your reading and writing skills.

Reading

Writing an essay requires knowledge of the topic, in part achieved through effective reading. Reading is critical to your success at university. Remember that it was common in the recent past for students to say that they were 'reading' a subject rather than 'studying' a subject at university; indeed, many still do. As the discussion on thinking above suggests, you cannot approach reading an academic text as you might a novel. There is a different purpose to academic reading and the manner in which you engage with the text requires you to be active in seeking meaning for learning to develop. There are also differences in language, structure and style. Unless you are an avid reader you will find the quantity you have to read increases and that what you read will change; in particular as your studies progress you will read more and more journal articles.

However, it is important that you continue to read a variety of texts in addition to academic works, including newspapers, magazines and novels. Research, for example that of Datta and MacDonald-Ross (2002), has shown that students who read frequently are more likely to have an enhanced vocabulary and are in a position to deal better with the demands and rigour of academic life, as are those who read more demanding works such as broadsheet newspapers, as opposed to the tabloids. This confirms our view in Chapter 2 of the importance of lexicon, for both your studies and practice.

It is a good idea for you to understand and think about your own reading habits as a foundation for developing strategies to enhance your skills.

ACTIVITY 3.5

Write down the name of the last novel you read, the last newspaper you read and the last magazine you read and when.

- Are these texts you typically read?

Now ask yourself: what would be a more difficult novel, newspaper or magazine for you to read? Get a copy of one of these and read it, reflecting on the experience. In particular make note of:

- your thoughts and feelings about reading something different;
- your experience of reading this text;
- what you understood and what you didn't understand;
- where and when you read.

Alternatively, read a piece of poetry and ask yourself the same questions as above.

Comment

There are common experiences when reading something different, particularly if the language and style are unfamiliar. It can make you think that you do not have the skills and knowledge to succeed; that you lack the intelligence required; you can easily become bored and distracted, or if you persevere the attendant feelings of frustration can come to the fore so that you misread and misinterpret the text. If this is the case you are in danger of reading, as discussed in Chapter 1, at a surface level, in which case you will gain some information but a limited understanding of the text. A deep understanding of the text requires you to become an active reader and to search for meaning consistently as you read.

A deep approach to reading

An important aspect of this is to consider the impact of the environment in which you are reading and whether or not this helps or hinders you. It is good to use the time and opportunity available to you to read so you may become accustomed to reading on the bus, for example. However, ask yourself if the environment is conducive to deep learning or to surface learning, since it is possible that having read a text on the bus, you need to revisit it in a different environment to engage fully with the meaning. A further element of deep reading is to establish how long you effectively read for and we recommend that you develop a habit of using several short periods of reading rather than one or two longer periods. Of course, the determination of how long exactly is subjective and will be different for each reader. It is necessary that you actively consider the impact that reading is having on your learning as you read – are you more or less fully engaged? If the latter, take a short break and perhaps do something else before returning to your text.

Reading with a purpose

A number of simple tasks are useful in establishing a deep approach to reading. This includes establishing the purpose for reading, that is, being as specific as possible about what you need from the text. The most obvious illustration of this is that you do not need to read a full book on developmental psychology to find out about cognitive development; you would go straight to the relevant section. Nonetheless, in reading the chapter or section on cognitive development you also need to appreciate what it is you are required to understand from the text and to take into consideration the issues discussed above in thinking about the literature.

It is also likely that you will come across unusual and unfamiliar words that impact upon the fluidity of your reading and your understanding of the text. Authors do not deliberately set out to make life difficult for a reader; however they do write with a particular readership in mind and do want to make sure that they engage that readership in terms of the discussion and argument and that the work is accepted as valid and worthwhile. The same author will take a different approach when writing about, for example, cognitive development for first-year undergraduates in an introductory textbook than when writing about the same topic in a peer-reviewed journal, that is, a journal that will be read by peers and other academics. When you do come across unfamiliar words it is helpful to have a dictionary at hand and whilst a standard dictionary will be useful you should also consider a subject-specific dictionary for some subjects. The language in sociology or in medical subjects, for example, can appear foreign and complicated and a sociology or medical dictionary will be invaluable. Also remember the importance of lexicon and the need to expand your own vocabulary, as discussed in Chapter 2.

Once you have understood what it is you are looking for it is a good idea to read the introduction or abstract and the conclusion to get an appreciation of whether or not the text is indeed useful. If so, you can read the text in full, particularly of a chapter in a book. You may be able to be more discerning in reading a journal article because many articles use a typical structure – abstract, introduction, literature review, methodology, findings, discussion and conclusion. If your purpose is simply to describe the findings of the research discussed in an article you may decide to skim over any consideration of the methodology used to carry out the research. However, if your purpose is to critically analyse then it is probable that you could find questions about the methodology useful in your analysis.

Reading notes

Many students will highlight parts of a text that they think are important or relevant and, particularly when new to a subject or a text, will find that they end up highlighting a lot of text. This is indicative of reading without discrimination and of not yet having established a deep approach to reading. In addition to highlighting, you should also consider writing (using a pencil) questions or thoughts in the margins that establish a query or understanding for why you have highlighted a particular sentence or words in the first instance. Therefore, even with highlighting, it will not be unusual to read something through for the first time and to feel that you have not fully understood the text. After your first read-through, make brief notes highlighting what you think the overall content has been about with specific reference to those elements that you have clearly understood. Likewise you should note those parts that you are not so clear about. Look at any queries or comments that you have made in the margins and question whether or not these agree with your notes. The next step is to reread the text, both to check your understanding and to develop your comprehension of those parts that were less clear. Remove from the margins any queries or comments that are now irrelevant or misinterpret the text.

The suggestions above reflect the SQ3R approach to reading and study:

Survey: Skim through the chapter or article and note the layout. Read the abstract, introduction and conclusion and note the themes. Look at the headings and other emphasis used in the text. Familiarise yourself with tables and charts.

Question: Look at the headings and ask questions about how the text is structured. Think about the questions you will need to keep in mind while reading and consider whether or not the book is relevant for your needs.

Read: With your questions in mind, read each section at a time. Consider whether your questions have been answered or if there are more questions. You might want to read through twice quickly.

Recall: Write down the main themes and issues discussed. If necessary, write your questions next to the relevant part of the text. The aim is to train yourself to answer the questions without reference to the text. It is essential to record the bibliographic details.

Review: Go over the questions again until you are sure that you have understood the text. If you have been taking notes, reread them to ensure their accuracy and to record any new ideas.

From reading to writing – referencing and plagiarism

Where there are elements of a text that you wish to use in your own work it is a good idea to make a note of the reference so that you can find the text when you need it but also to help you to organise a citation within your own work or to complete your bibliography or reference list on completion of an essay. Acknowledging another person's work is an absolute requirement within academic assessments and not to do so risks allegations of plagiarism and of cheating.

Plagiarism occurs when you use someone else's work and claim it as your own. This can happen inadvertently, because you have not cited the work properly or at all, or because you think it is acceptable to cheat. It is very easy, particularly given the amount of information available on the internet and the ease of 'cut and paste', to manipulate text and to use it within your own work. You should remember that plagiarism committed inadvertently is still an offence. Increasingly tutors and universities are asking students to submit work electronically through plagiarism detection software to halt the possibility of cheating. Minor findings of plagiarism are likely to result in students having to redo their assessment. However, the most serious case can result in a student's studies being terminated.

One of the most useful ways to avoid plagiarism is to record and organise your references in an index card system. These can either be paper-based or electronic and they allow you to store information based on author or topic. It is important that the card contains two types of information – the reference that will properly cite the work and an annotation or brief description of the text. A card for this chapter would contain information similar to this:

Oko, J and Reid, J (2012) *Study Skills for Health and Social Care Students.* London: Sage.

Chapter 3
The discussion covers using ICT to find literature, how to think about the literature and then how to use this within an assessment. Particularly important to remember planning and preparation and to read regularly.

There are a number of referencing systems in use and you need to make sure that you are using the one required by your university or tutor. The most common are the Vancouver or endnote system and the Harvard system. In the former, citations are given a number in the order in which they appear in the text. If this system was used in this book then the citations in this chapter would appear as Goleman (1) or as a superscript number, Bruce,[2] and so forth. Depending on the particular requirements of your tutor or university, the full reference would then appear in numerical order as a footnote and/or a list of references at the end of your text.

The Harvard system, used throughout this book, is an author, date, alphabetic system where the name of the authors and date of publication appear in the body of the text and the full reference is given within an alphabetical list at the end of the text. Just look at the examples all through this book. The following illustrations cover only a few of the important Harvard conventions; you need to make sure that you become familiar with the guidance provided by your tutors and university.

When citing the work of another within your text using the Harvard system there are a number of requirements. When you are using the name of the author within your sentence you need to put the date in brackets:

Reid (2007) develops the idea that assessments are flawed.

or

Oko and Reid (2012) consider planning and preparation as essential to successful study.

Where there are more than two authors you can use:

Oko et al. (2010).

If you are not using the author's name within your sentence it is necessary to do the following:

Poor understanding of theory is a contributory factor to poor assessments (Reid, 2007).

or:

Deficits in assessment are predicted without proper planning and preparation (Oko and Reid, 2012).

If you use a quotation, the same conventions apply but it is also necessary to include the page number of the original work where the quotation can be found, to use the exact words and punctuation and to use quotation marks.

Poor understanding of theory is 'a contributory factor to poor assessments' (Reid, 2007, p25).

When constructing a full reference at the end of your work there are again conventions to follow depending on how the original work was published.

Books

Oko, J (2011) *Understanding and Using Theory in Social Work* (2nd edition). Exeter: Learning Matters.

Notice that the name of the book is in italics and that the place of publication is written before the name of the publisher. In addition, references are always presented in alphabetical order.

Chapters in a book

Reid, J (2007) Developing inclusive practice in children and families social work, in Tovey, W (ed) *The Post-Qualifying Handbook for Social Workers.* London: Jessica Kingsley Publishers.

The author's name and the date are given followed by the title of the chapter. As this is an edited book the name of the editor is then provided followed by the title of the book in italics. Finally the publisher's details are given.

Journals

Reid, J (2007) To register or not – the relevance of the social work codes of practice for the social work lecturer. *Ethics and Social Welfare,* 1 (3): 336–341.

In this illustration the title of the article is in sentence case (starting with a capital letter) and the name of the journal is in italics. The numbers after the name of the journal refer to volume 1, issue 3 and the relevant page numbers.

Websites

The conventions on referencing websites are continuing to develop and again you should check with your tutor and university exactly how they want this done. However the basic elements remain:

Social Care Institute for Excellence (SCIE) (2009) *Communication Skills [online].* Available: www.scie.org.uk/publications/elearning/cs/index.asp [accessed 16 November 2009]

It is important to give the date that you accessed the webpage as the information can change over time.

ACTIVITY 3.6

It is a good idea to practise writing references. Choose a book with a single author, an edited book (one with many contributors), an academic journal and a website and write a reference for each using the Harvard system.

Hint: if you are unsure, look at the referencing within the text you are reading.

Writing

Proper citations and referencing are just some of the conventions that you are expected to use in your writing at university. Other expectations include the proper use of English, involving minimal errors in spelling, punctuation, grammar and syntax. There are some basic points to bear in mind from the outset.

- Spell checkers are helpful but only if you are using the correct version. This means using the UK English and not US English version.
- There is no substitute for reading over your work more than once. Many basic errors can be eliminated by effective proofreading. This can include asking someone else to read your work before submission (you can have a reciprocal arrangement with someone else in your class). It should include reading your work out loud to yourself; hearing what you have written will overcome those internal notions that you have about your work. Often, awkward or nonsensical sentences can be detected by listening to them.
- Syntax is the systematic and grammatical use of words in a sentence and you need to understand the rules of grammar to write coherent and interesting essays. Think about the need to reduce sentences that are too long into shorter more meaningful ones. New paragraphs are useful when discussing different ideas or points.
- Good punctuation is required and should not be ignored. The BBC Skillswise website offers helpful fact sheets on grammar and punctuation: **www.bbc.co.uk/skillswise/ english**.
- Avoid colloquialisms and writing as you speak. For example, it is: *he should* have *recorded the information immediately* and not *he should* of *recorded the information immediately*.
- Before you write, plan (see Activity 3.1 and below).
- Write in an environment that is conducive to writing. Use a comfortable chair and sit at a desk or table that is the correct height. Try to avoid distractions.
- Understand the question and any instructions provided, paying particular attention to the marking criteria. Additionally, be careful to follow any instructions provided by your tutor in relation to word length, word allocation and style. Typically you will not be penalised for writing ten per cent under or over the set word limit but you may be if you use too many or too little words in a particular section.
- Make sure you understand from which viewpoint you are writing. Some essays are written in the third person, for example if you were analysing Piaget's theory of cognitive development (e.g. he proposed that . . .). Others will be written in the first person, such as an analysis of how you put into practice Piaget's theory of cognitive development (e.g. I established that . . .).

The writing process

Committing your first words to paper can be a daunting task as you strive to meet all diverse expectations and for many novice students the experience can be overwhelming. However by adopting the following steps, you will be able to approach writing with more clarity and less stress.

- Planning. Begin by developing a mind map with the question in the centre of the map. Get all of the ideas you want to use down on paper in this diagrammatical form and number each in the order that you want to use them in your essay. Remember that a plan is not set in stone: you can develop it and adapt it as you write your essay. Through effective planning and preparation you can overcome many of the pitfalls and behaviours that make essay-writing difficult. Much of the planning and preparation includes activities we have already covered in this chapter – understanding the question, and in particular the words used to define the thinking skills you are required to demonstrate, providing sufficient time to complete the task and reading and rereading key texts.

- Drafting. An essay has three basic elements to it – introduction, main body and conclusion. The main body is the substantive part of the essay and is developed from your plan. Remember to leave writing your introduction to the end as it is easier to introduce what you have already written rather than change an already written introduction. As you write your draft, continually refer back to the question and to the plan to check that you are maintaining focus. A draft is a long way from being a final submission, so never be defeated by a blank page. It is better to write something and to review it later and change it than to waste time battling with nothing. The conclusion should summarise the main body of the essay succinctly and accurately. Do not develop new ideas in your conclusion and always make sure you have answered the question.

- Editing. There are many anecdotes of students who leave their essay-writing to the last possible minute and who lose marks, not necessarily because their ideas are wrong but because they ran out of time to proofread, develop and restructure to ensure the fluidity of their argument. Editing also involves making sure that the presentation of the essay is of the necessary standard. You may be required to use a particular font, font size and spacing between lines. Ensure that there are spaces between paragraphs and that the pages are numbered. Check that your reference list and/or bibliography is included and provide a cover page if necessary.

- Use feedback. Other people are a useful resource in the development of ideas; you can bounce ideas off friends and family or ask them for feedback about something you have written. You can also use tutors in this way. At the outset it is important to bear in mind that it is unlikely you will get everything right every time. Learning includes the capacity to make mistakes and to develop new knowledge from this. A critical component of this process is the feedback you receive from tutors who make suggestions about how to develop your work. (Look back to the case study of Anna in Chapter 1, Activity 1.2.) The feedback provided by tutors is meant to add to your ability to reflect on the weaknesses and strengths of your skills and knowledge, thus allowing you to think about how you might improve and progress. Crucially it is not necessary to wait until you hand your work in to receive feedback as there will be opportunities to do so before final submission. Comments offered on work that you have handed in to be marked are known as 'summative' feedback; however, comments offered on work in progress, such as a draft of an essay, are known as 'formative' feedback and this is an effective way for you to check your progress. Moreover the availability of formative feedback is an encouragement to get on with the task.

Difficulties with reading and writing

Some students will require additional support with reading because of a learning difficulty such as dyslexia or dyspraxia. Dyslexia is the impairment of reading skills regardless of intelligence and dyslexic adults may avoid reading, be slow to read, rely on verbal rather than reading skills, have poor spelling and appear disorganised. Dyspraxia can affect fine motor skills and writing or typing may be impaired. It is still possible that many people reach adulthood without a diagnosis; however neither dyslexia nor dyspraxia should be a barrier to successful study. Students who know or think they are dyslexic or dyspraxic should seek an assessment of their learning needs within the university. These are undertaken by trained staff who, with your agreement and where necessary, will inform tutors of the impact of the condition on your learning and what steps to take to support you in your learning. It is important to remember that you need to be proactive in seeking such an assessment.

PART TWO SUMMARY

- Consider the SQ3R approach to reading and study – survey, question, read, recall, review – as a method for actively reading a text.
- An active engagement with the text is necessary in order to read purposively, develop a deep understanding of the text and help in generating your own ideas and new knowledge.
- You will use the work of others within your own work, so it is crucial that you become accustomed to citations and referencing. We recommend that you get into the habit of noting annotated references as you read.
- The capacity to reference correctly stands alongside the good use of English and good presentation as key components in supporting the coherence of your argument and the reader's ability to understand it.
- Good essays will develop from good planning and preparation followed by a draft that is edited and reviewed.
- You should use the feedback provided by tutors to develop your future written work.

Chapter 4 continues the theme of communication skill enhancement by focusing on developing effective presentation skills.

FURTHER READING

Burnard, P (2004) *Writing Skills in Health Care.* Cheltenham: Nelson Thornes.
A straightforward and easy-to-use book that is suitable for novice writers and those returning to studies after a break.

Gregor, C (2006) *Practical Computer Skills for Social Work.* Exeter: Learning Matters.
This book covers the range of IT skills necessary for successful study. It begins with a learning needs profile to identify your strengths and areas for improvement. It will be helpful to practitioners from all professions.

Healy, K and Mullholland, J (2007) *Writing Skills for Social Workers.* London: Sage.
A practical and engaging book that considers professional writing skills as well as those necessary for study.

http://learnhigher.ac.uk/Students/Information-literacy.html
Learn Higher: this website has lots of helpful information and exercises to help students develop their ICT skills. It provides a definition of information literacy and references the SCONUL seven pillars.

4 DEVELOPING PRESENTATION SKILLS

CHAPTER OBJECTIVES

By the end of this chapter you should be able to:

- understand the purpose of presentations both as an applied professional task and in academic life;

- appreciate the need for good planning, preparation and practice and recognise a variety of approaches that you can adopt to overcome anxiety and to develop good presentations;

- develop your awareness of your existing presentational skills and how to enhance these.

Introduction

Presentations are commonly used in both your studies and in professional life; nonetheless the act of standing up in front of a group of people and speaking can give rise to fear and anxiety. This can be exacerbated if the purpose of the presentation is an assessment of your knowledge and skills, a job interview or when you need to convince others to provide a service or resources for someone in need. The good news is that such reactions are not unusual and it is possible with planning, preparation and practice to become a competent and persuasive speaker. Just as in Chapter 3, where you were introduced to a few steps that can help you develop your written work, there are practical steps to follow to achieve a coherent and successful presentation. As you might appreciate, you should expect to spend time and effort before your presentation both to help deal with any anxiety and to meet the purpose of the presentation. Not to do so risks a poor assessment outcome, not getting the job or, of vital importance to the most vulnerable in society, not receiving a service or resources. Presentational skills are not only required as a means of demonstrating understanding in the classroom context but also represent a key skill in professional practice.

Are you an experienced presenter?

Before we begin this section complete Activity 4.1.

ACTIVITY 4.1
This should take 15 minutes to complete. Think about the times you have had to do presentations in the past and list:

- the purpose of the presentation;
- who the presentation was made to;
- any tools used, for example, flip charts, posters, PowerPoint.

From your list you may be surprised at the number of times you have been involved in presenting in the past; indeed, if your list includes only a few examples you are probably underestimating your presenting history and you have perhaps concentrated on formal types of presentation, for example, as an assessment to tutors. Formal presentations are perhaps more memorable to you because they are associated with heightened levels of anxiety. This is because, in addition to saying the right thing, you are concerned with achieving a highly refined performance. The danger here is that the message may get lost in preference to the desire to look good – an approach that Anna in the case study from Chapter 1 might adopt if she were giving a presentation. However, the primary purpose of presentations must be to communicate the message: a polished performance is good but should not be the most important element.

The difference can be seen when you consider the range of informal presentations you undertake. We often use informal presentations to provide a quick and convenient overview of ideas or issues, such as when sketching out an idea on paper or whiteboard to a small group of peers. On these occasions you are attempting to communicate an idea to the listeners and you are concentrating on getting the message across. You are not as anxious in these situations because they are an extension of a conversation with your listeners; you are talking to rather than at them. When you take into consideration informal situations you can recognise that presentations are a much more common feature of your interaction with others, particularly if you remember that presentations are purposefully used as an effective tool in conveying information to another person or groups of people. They are employed to give information, instruct, persuade, influence and/or to entertain. Some presentations may do only one of these, some may encompass them all but whatever their purpose, presentations are essentially about communication and not performance.

ACTIVITY 4.2
Look at Figure 4.1. Read it once or twice and, without hesitating, give a presentation lasting at least one minute using the topics included.

> • Mobile phone
>
> • Text and email and tweets
>
> • iPod or MP3
>
> • Microsoft Windows and Internet Explorer

Figure 4.1 **Information technologies**

The presentation process

You were able to complete this activity because you are familiar with the content and you already possess a range of communication skills. If you think again about the number of times that you have had to give information, instruct, persuade, influence or even entertain in the informal sense, you should be able to expand upon your original list in Activity 4.1. This also reinforces the fact that you have some skills and knowledge in undertaking presentations and they are simply a tool to be used from your experience to enhance your existing communication skills. The good news is we can all communicate and the variety of tools to support our communication is developing all the time, with electronic aids such as PowerPoint, Twitter and Facebook now very common; nonetheless the underlying processes and approaches are the same.

- At the outset you define the purpose or aim. What do you need to communicate, for what purpose and to whom?
- Knowing yourself and your audience helps when deciding on the means and content of communication. Checking your assumptions about the audience includes consideration of the language or images to be used and the strengths and limitations of the medium for the presentation.
- Getting the information across and being heard. You need to consider timing and to make sure that the technology works or is accessible. There is no point in using a flip chart if you have no pen or using electronic methods of communication if the recipient cannot access the message. The content of the communication should match the intended message.
- Recipient and reciprocal processing. Remember that once you have communicated something, this has to be received and processed by the recipient. Pacing is important and the more information there is, the longer such processing may take. Your understanding of what you have said or shown may not be what has been understood. You are also active in receiving non-verbal cues back from those to whom you are presenting.
- Checking understanding. Clarity and space for questions are always welcome and can set aside some of the assumptions you have made about the recipients and their understanding during the communication.
- Review. Receiving feedback and evaluating the presentation are crucial to developing your skills and to learning.

Good presentations are within all of your capabilities and you are all practised communicators. With time and effort, you can enhance your prospects both within your studies and in your professional life. We will now consider the importance of presentations for the helping professional.

Why are presentations necessary?

The Quality Assurance Agency (QAA) for Higher Education determines the qualities, knowledge and skills required to achieve the status of graduate in the UK. Graduates are able to *communicate information, ideas, problems and solutions to both specialist and non-specialist audiences* and holders of UK degrees *will have the qualities and transferrable skills necessary for employment* (Quality Assurance Agency, 2008, p19), which of course include the ability and skill to communicate effectively. In addition the 'Dublin descriptors', which describe the generic and common features of graduateness across Europe, include a communication skills element reflected in the QAA statement above. The QAA also produces a series of subject benchmark statements designed to illuminate and qualify the nature of graduateness in particular subjects and for programmes of qualification for the helping professions. Each of the statements includes specific reference to communication, including the ability to search and retrieve information and to interpret and present information using a variety of media.

Professional and regulatory bodies are also concerned to ensure skilful and competent communication, as the following examples illustrate:

- Nursing and Midwifery Council Code: *Standards of conduct, performance and ethics for nurses and midwives* (2008) includes a requirement to share with people, in a way they can understand, the information they want or need to know about their health.
- General Social Care Council (GSCC) *Codes of Practice for Social Care Workers* (2010), including social workers, includes the requirement to communicate in an appropriate, open, accurate and straightforward way.
- The Health Professions Council (2008) *Standards of Conduct, Performance and Ethics* (**www.hpc-uk.org/publications/standards**) require you to communicate properly and effectively with service users and other practitioners.
- The *Professional and National Occupational Standards for Youth Work* (National Youth Agency, 2008) require youth workers to communicate effectively and develop rapport with young people.
- Not only are professional and regulatory bodies concerned with the need for effective communication, governments have also endorsed this as a key area of competence, for example the Department of Children, Schools and Families' *Common Core of Skills and Knowledge for the Children's Workforce* states that:

Good communication is central to working with [people] . . . It is important to be able to communicate both on a one-on-one basis and in a group context. Communication is not just about the words you use, but also your manner of speaking, body language and, above all, the effectiveness with which you listen. To communicate effectively it is important to take account of culture and context, for example where English is an additional language.

(HM Government, 2005, p6)

Good communication and the willingness and ability to develop and deliver effective presentations are much more than a vehicle for educational assessment, although this is an important facet of their use; they are also crucial to achieving positive outcomes for those with whom you work. Good communication, including the ability to present effectively, is a transferable skill, that is, it can be used in many different situations or contexts. So the skills that you learn and develop in university or college you will be able to take with you into your later work role and thus be better placed to offer an effective service to those you are working with. A professional approach to your work also moves beyond meeting standards to include personal attitudes, values and beliefs. The term 'professional' denotes someone who is knowledgeable, articulate and qualified but it also signifies ethical behaviour. As a student undertaking a course leading to a qualification in one of the helping professions, you will be expected to adopt a professional approach to your studies and to apply yourself to a range of tasks that are part of the competent practitioner's repertoire, including, of course, presentations.

Planning and preparing your presentation

Planning, preparation and practice are essential for a good presentation and are core components of competent professional practice. In Activity 4.1 above you learned that you have used presentations on many occasions and, although there are different types of presentation, their primary purpose is communication. You may have to communicate individually or as a member of a group; you may be expected to use a particular technology such as PowerPoint or to design a poster and the presentation may be formal or informal. Whatever the context or purpose, there are a number of questions to take into account that will help achieve a good outcome. Before we consider these questions more fully, complete Activity 4.3.

ACTIVITY 4.3

Imagine you are applying for a place on a course at university that leads to a professional qualification in one of the helping professions. The selection process requires you to undertake a ten-minute presentation using slides or PowerPoint. The title of the presentation is:

'Why this course is good for me and why I am good for this course.'

- Write down your immediate thoughts about the content of this presentation.
- Develop a plan for this presentation, thinking about the number of slides and their likely content.
- What questions did you consider in developing your plan?

Comment

In completing this exercise you will have thought of a number of key things that you want to communicate to the interviewers and made decisions and assumptions about the purpose and potential content of the presentation. Some of the points you need to include may appear more obvious than others and you will have spent longer thinking about some than others. Your initial consideration of content could include:

- knowledge of the course curriculum;
- knowledge of the professional role;
- any experience you have;
- recent issues perhaps discussed in the media involving your chosen area of practice;
- your attributes, knowledge and skills.

This is not an exhaustive list but the content is typical and now you will begin to think about the structure of the presentation, including the content of the PowerPoint slides.

Stop!

Although you are likely to have come up with some relevant ideas about content, it is important that you do not assume that you have. It is also essential to take time to allow other ideas and issues to develop. Achieving a good outcome requires you to spend time planning your presentation and there are a number of essential questions that will help you to decide both content and structure and reassure you that you understand what and why you are presenting what you are.

What is the purpose of the presentation?

This might appear obvious but you can too easily dismiss this question and misjudge the focus. As with an essay question, a presentation has an aim: in the case of Activity 4.3 this could be: to convince the interviewers that you have the necessary qualities and attributes to undertake their course and to demonstrate that you understand the professional purpose and content of the course. Whatever aim you define, it is important to use a verb that is specific and achievable, such as, to convince, to inform, to illustrate, to explain, to describe.

> ### ACTIVITY 4.4
> It is helpful to state the aim of the presentation in a single sentence. Now write an aim for your presentation, described in Activity 4.3.

Comment

In addition to stating an explicit aim, you may need to consider the elements necessary to achieving your aim – these are known as objectives. Objectives are usually written from an evaluation point of view and may contain aspects of behaviour or quantity. They are also commonly set out following a trunk or part of a sentence, for example:

By the end of this presentation the interviewers will be able to:

- understand the knowledge, qualities and skills that demonstrate my potential as a good student (behaviour);
- describe the six key attributes that I will bring to this course as a student (quantity).

As with your aim, your objectives should be achievable and realistic. They should also be relevant to your aim; there is nothing to be gained by discussing your personal qualities or the skills you have gained through hobbies or voluntary work if you do not explicitly link these to the purpose of the presentation.

> **ACTIVITY 4.5**
> Think about your objectives for the presentation outlined in Activity 4.3 and write a
> trunk list of your objectives.

Defining the aim and objectives is the first step in deciding on the structure of the presentation. As you now know what you want to communicate to your listeners, you will almost immediately begin to think of how best to communicate this; there are, however other important questions to consider before moving on to this.

Who will be listening to my presentation?

Good communication requires you to engage with your listeners and thus you need to understand their purpose in listening to you. This requires consideration of their concerns and priorities and, importantly for the helping professions, what their values are. In an interview for social work, nursing and similar courses you are likely to encounter a panel of at least two people, a tutor from the course and a practitioner currently working in the field of study. It helps to remember that many course tutors have also been practitioners in the past or indeed may continue to practise in some capacity. For some courses you may also be interviewed by service users. If it is not clear from the outset you should try to find out who will be involved in the interview panel. Once you know this you will be able to discern the differences in their focus and priorities. Completing Activity 4.6 will help you to understand this.

> **ACTIVITY 4.6**
> Courses leading to a qualification in the helping professions inevitably have three
> important components – knowledge, values and skills. Assuming that there will be two
> people involved in listening to your presentation, a tutor and a practitioner, under the
> headings knowledge, values and skills, list the priorities you think each will have.

Activity 4.6 points to another essential aspect of planning and preparation – the need to undertake some research. For this activity it is necessary that you know of the knowledge, values and skills required by your chosen profession as these are central to the learning and teaching strategies and curriculum adopted by the course. The same would be true if the presentation had a different focus. For example, if you were asked to 'describe the range of factors that may lead to atypical development in early childhood' you would need to research early child development; factors affecting development such as poverty; alcohol and drug misuse; disability, and so on. In the interview example it might immediately appear that the knowledge, values and skills are common for the tutor and the practitioner; however they may emphasise different sides of the same coin as both will bring their own views, values and interests to the interview. Both will want you to communicate your potential as a learner and as a future practitioner; the tutor may concentrate on the former and the practitioner on the latter. Where you are able to talk about practical experience within your presentation, the tutor may focus on what you learned from this experience and the practitioner on the practical skills you have developed. The tutor may be interested in your knowledge of the curriculum, the practitioner in your knowledge of policies and processes used in practice, and so forth. Whatever focus you decide upon, it is necessary that you take account of those who will be listening to your presentation.

How do I engage the listeners?

Just as understanding the priorities and values of the listeners is important in engagement, so is your understanding of the use of body language and other tools. Non-verbal communication is discussed in Chapter 2; however it is worth reiterating some important points.

- Appearance is important so dress suitably for the context.
- Smile and say hello.
- Introduce yourself and maintain eye contact with all the listeners, not just one.
- Use small, open gestures for emphasis and avoid those that are distracting.
- If you are part of a group presentation, actively listen when other group members are presenting.
- Speak clearly and without rushing.

It is important that you get your pitch, tone and pace right to keep an audience interested. A speaker who cannot be heard or is too loud, who speaks in a monotone or whose delivery is too quick or too slow will not communicate effectively with the listeners and will fail to convey the message. Ask your listeners if they can hear you, especially those sitting further back, and try to keep your head up when you speak as this aids eye contact and means that your voice is being directed outwards and not to the floor. You should try not to read directly from a script but use your notes or cue cards as an aide-mémoire only. Choose your words and language carefully and try to avoid jargon and 'ums' and 'ers'; colloquial language could be perceived as unprofessional.

You will be able to tell from the listeners' body language whether or not they are actively listening to you; using your voice effectively by varying pitch, tone and pace will help to maintain listener interest. The majority of inexperienced presenters will speak too fast as a result of nerves, so there is work to be done in preparing your voice prior to the presentation. Although it may seem foolish or give rise to feelings of embarrassment, the adage that 'practice makes perfect' should be heeded. Once you have completed your presentation, stand in front of a mirror and practise, deliver your presentation to friends or family or to the other members of your group and take heed of their feedback. Listen to your voice by recording it; listening back to yourself will bring to light aspects of your speaking style of which you are not aware, commonly the repeated use of a favoured word or inflection. The embarrassment you feel at practising will be nothing to what you would feel if your presentation does not go to plan. Practice is also an effective measure of whether or not you have timed your presentation correctly.

You will engage your listeners by taking into consideration their needs and by treating them with respect; you will talk to them and not at them. Planning, preparation and practice will ensure that your time and theirs is not wasted and you should also offer them the opportunity to talk to you by allowing time for questions or feedback. This may appear daunting but if you have taken the time to consider the questions and exercises above you will be well prepared for questions. Remember that honesty is important and that sometimes saying 'I don't know' is the correct answer.

How should I structure my presentation?

Presentations are similar to essays in that they should have an introduction, a main body and a conclusion; however the similarities end there. When reading an article or a book the reader is able to go back over previous sections or information that has some bearing on what is currently being read, but this is not possible with a presentation and it is important that you keep together all of the relevant elements of your discussion. In the presentation outlined in Activity 4.3 you should not, for example, discuss your experiences as a learner in your previous educational setting and then return to this theme some minutes later. This will only cause the listener to lose focus. McCarthy and Hatcher (2002, pp72–74) discuss a number of possible patterns that can be used to structure a presentation depending on the aim and objectives identified earlier:

- Chronological – good when you need to depict development over a period of time. Limits discussion of issues that are outside your chronology or timeline.
- Spatial – good when relating points to a range of places, for example, the differences in approach to an issue adopted by the UK, France and Sweden.
- Causal – your views of the causes of an issue dealt with in turn.
- Topical – stating the important aspects, in consideration of a particular question or issue, in turn.
- Theory and practice – the theory or hypothesis behind a situation is given and then related to practice (or vice versa).
- Problem and solution – the content is organised to look at a presenting problem and a solution to it.

With this in mind complete Activity 4.7.

ACTIVITY 4.7

Prepare a structure for the presentation outlined in Activity 4.3. Remember that you only have ten minutes and draw upon the results of the activities already undertaken.

Comment

It is probable that you will decide to use a topical pattern for this presentation. How you order your topics will depend on your experiences, interests and issues you want to emphasise; nonetheless you should conform to the requirement for an introduction, a main body and a conclusion. Before presenting your topics you should ensure that your introduction is sufficient to get your listeners' attention, to gain their interest and to establish the correct pitch and tone for the environment. Sometimes it can help to begin with a brief anecdote or joke just to get everyone listening before sketching the main body of the presentation. If you are part of a group presentation it is possible that someone has already done this before you, and on such occasions you could make reference to the previous presenter, thus reinforcing the continuity between the different contributions.

Just as the presentation overall has a beginning, middle and end, so can individual slides, particularly those in the main body of the presentation, but this will be of no use if you fail to consider a few simple points: keep the style (background, font, font size, colour) consistent; make sure that colours enhance the presentation and that you can read the slides; keep animation and sound to a minimum, and only use if essential; use images to illustrate but try not to place text over them; use the templates provided. Having settled on the style of the slide you can turn your attention to the content, detailed in Figure 4.2.

Beginning: each slide should have a heading or title that captures the main issues to be discussed. A font size larger than the main body should be used

Main body:

- bullet point one

- bullet point two

- bullet point three

- bullet point four

Each bullet point is a synopsis of a point you want to make. You should refer to each in turn and elaborate on the meaning and relevance of the point being raised. Note that slides should not contain too much information; they are an aid to your speech and listeners should not be distracted from looking at you by reading the slides. Nor should you simply read the slides; you need to expand on each bullet point.

Figure 4.2 **Presentation slides**

The conclusion is not normally displayed on the slide but requires you, where necessary, to summarise one slide and link it to the next, providing continuity throughout the presentation.

Delivering your presentation – dealing with nerves and anxiety

Feeling nervous or anxious before a presentation is common. It is an indication that you want the presentation to go well but that you are perhaps fearful of the unknown, of making a mistake, of being judged, of not being able to answer a question, and so forth. In these situations your body responds by releasing adrenaline which makes your heart pump faster, your lungs breathe quicker to supply more oxygen and, as your body heats up, you sweat to cool down. However your mind becomes more focused and for this final reason some anxiety can be a good thing, particularly if you can learn to harness this enhanced concentration.

You can begin to do this by asking yourself whether your fears about the presentation are rational. Where you have had a negative experience in the past, think also of the occasions that were successful and more enjoyable. There is always more than one way of considering an experience and it is important to begin by thinking positively and to remember that, with proper preparation and planning, you will know the content of the presentation and will have greatly lessened the likelihood of any mishaps. You may also have higher expectations of yourself than the listeners who are unlikely to expect perfection and will tolerate mistakes. Your mind set when presenting should be to accept mistakes as a normal constituent in presentations, not dwelling on any mistakes but moving on. You can do this either by maintaining the integrity of the presentation and moving to the next point or by using it as an opportunity for a pause, to gather your thoughts, to make a joke at your own expense. Being able to pause to regain your thoughts is admired more by listeners than someone who muddles through. It is a sign of confidence and of concern to ensure that the message of the presentation is communicated and is respectful to the listeners.

> ### REFLECTION POINT
> Think about yourself standing in front of a group of peers and tutors about to make a presentation. How do you imagine you may be feeling? What is your body's response to this situation? Write your answers down.

Have a look at your list and decide which fears are rational and think how you might deal with them. The following points will also help but remember that you can and should also talk to your tutor if you think you are unable to deal with this alone.

- We have noted that you are already a practised communicator and a good place to begin your preparation for any presentation is to think about your strengths and the requirements for effective communication, discussed in Chapter 2. Do not allow your esteem to be overpowered by irrational fears or thoughts. This can lead to a lack of confidence which in turn will affect how you think, feel, behave and present yourself physically.

You need to recognise your body's physiological response to the presentation situation and to take control of it by controlling your breathing and achieving a relaxed posture.

- Find a quiet space, free of disruptions, to close your eyes and to concentrate on your breathing. Take deep breaths into your lungs: you will recognise this because your stomach will rise as you inhale and deflate as you exhale. Over a number of minutes focus on exhaling and slow your breathing.

Slowing your breathing has the effect of decreasing the amount of adrenaline in your body.

Breathing exercises are an effective way of relaxing which can be further enhanced by dealing with any tightness in your body. If you are aware that certain parts of your body are tense, for example your shoulders, stretch and exercise them to release the tension.

- One way of doing this is to tense your muscles and then release when exhaling. Tense and release on an outward breath several times until the tension diminishes. Repeat as necessary for other areas of your body. Even if you do not feel tense it may help you to work your way up through your body, starting with your toes, and tensing and relaxing your main muscles.

Appearing relaxed to the listeners is important in developing rapport but it is also important to your own physical well-being and enjoyment of the experience.

You will also be aware of other techniques or rituals that you have developed to help you relax, for example, listening to music. Try to incorporate these into your preparation and develop a strategy that you follow prior to presentations. As part of this, think about your initial engagement with the listeners, remember the importance of eye contact and of a smile and a 'hello'. You may wish to use an anecdote to get you going – something like an amusing story or a reference from the news that is relevant to your presentation. This gives you time to gather your thoughts, is an effective introduction and allows the listeners time to concentrate on you without missing any of the substantive content of the presentation. In summary:

- use breathing exercises to lessen your anxieties and to become aware of tensions in your body;
- deal with tension by tensing and relaxing your muscles;
- following your breathing exercises use the adrenaline positively for enhanced concentration and focus;
- think positively and set aside irrational fears; remind yourself of your strengths and accomplishments;
- mistakes will happen; move on, the listeners don't expect perfection; what feels like an enormous problem to you probably isn't to those listening;
- you have prepared and practised, so maintain an even pace to keep in control.

Other types of presentation

This chapter has mainly focused on a presentation example that involves the use of PowerPoint because this will be familiar to the majority of you. There are other formats for presentations often used in universities and colleges, including the use of posters. Whatever the format used, the approaches outlined in this chapter in terms of knowing yourself, planning, preparation and practice still apply.

Poster presentations, as the name suggests, use a single 'sheet' to convey a clear message through the images and minimal text. The poster also serves to raise points of discussion between the presenter and viewer and so usually involves a more intimate conversation. The aims and objectives of the poster presentation should be conveyed clearly, as should the main points for discussion. Good posters should be focused and use images (not text) to convey meaning and should have an obvious sequence. Many posters are designed around a prominent or main image that is visually arresting and is used to gain the interest of the viewer. A poster may also require a different range of resources than those already available through PowerPoint so you need to consider if you have the required pictures, glue, pens and other related material. If you think that you have too much detail to cover than can be included in your poster, provide a handout.

You can also expect to be asked to present as a member of a group and there are some key points worth emphasising. A successful group presentation will depend on collaboration, organisation and explicitly stated expectations. It is helpful to decide upon a group leader to facilitate decisions about who is focusing on what part of the presentation; timing and order; format of slides, including colour and font; and, importantly, what the group members will do to show support and interest when not presenting. Of course group presentations can bring challenges that do not arise for a single presenter. Before any decisions about the presentation are made, the group will have to ensure that they function as a team, including taking into account any contingencies such as someone drying up or someone not turning up.

As you might expect, practice is essential to a coherent, fluid and meaningful group presentation. Not only is it important to rehearse timings but to ensure smooth transition from one presenter to the next, including introducing the next presenter. Groups should also consider introducing all members of the group at the outset.

CHAPTER SUMMARY

- Presentations are both an academic and an applied professional task.
- To complete them successfully requires appropriate planning, preparation and practice; not to do so risks a disservice to you and to those you are working with and presenting to.
- Taking into account the following key points will enhance your existing presentational skills:

   1. Know yourself – know your strengths and work to them.
   2. Define the aim and objectives of the presentation.
   3. Know your audience and take account of their priorities and values.
   4. Research your topic and get the most up-to-date information.
   5. Structure your presentation and slides with an introduction, main body and conclusion.
   6. Keep your slides simple and readable; animation and sound can be distracting but carefully chosen images can be useful.
   7. Use your voice effectively and use other communication skills to engage your listeners.
   8. Practise, practise, practise and ensure that any necessary equipment is in place and works. Consider a back-up such as handouts just in case.
   9. Keep to time.
   10. Leave time for questions or feedback.

In Chapter 5 we move on to consider the importance of practice learning and of preparation for this central part of your professional development.

FURTHER READING

Chivers, B and Shoolbred, M (2007) *A Student's Guide to Presentations: Making your presentation count.* London: Sage.
This book gives readers a detailed guide to the preparation and delivery of both individual and group presentations and takes you through all the practical stages necessary to complete a presentation and obtain excellent marks.

McCarthy, P and Hatcher, C (2002) *Presentation Skills: The essential guide for students.* London: Sage.
This is a well-written book that uses a step-by-step approach to enable you to gain in confidence and develop your approach to presentations. A good resource for those wanting to improve their skills.

5 PRACTICE LEARNING AND ETHICAL PRACTICE

CHAPTER OBJECTIVES

By the end of this chapter you should be able to:

- identify the professional and regulatory requirements necessary for competent practice;

- understand that ethical principles underpin good outcomes for service users and patients;

- identify skills for employability, including those that require enhancement.

Introduction

Many university and college courses offer the opportunity of practice learning or undertaking a placement. In this chapter we use the term 'practice learning' to denote a practice placement or clinical placement and to emphasise that such opportunities are also intrinsically part of your learning. Practice learning is seen as essential preparation for your future career and is much more than work experience. In professions working with people the emphasis in placement is on assessment of competence but also learning about those with whom you work, both service users or patients and colleagues, and about yourself. Practice learning culminates in assessment of knowledge, skills and values and a judgment by qualified, experienced peers and tutors of your competence and attainment against the required national occupational standards for your area of practice. It is an opportunity for you to show your critical understanding of your academic learning and how you apply this to your practice and continuing development.

The skills discussed throughout this book are wholly relevant to practice and will help you to demonstrate your abilities as a good practitioner. The chapters up to now have focused on skills that support good learning and also help to achieve good outcomes for people with whom you work. The final chapter will help you to think about your practice and to develop the critically reflective approach that is the backbone of continuing professional development and good outcomes. You should seek to enhance the skills discussed throughout this book prior to placement and continue to refer to the book throughout your practice learning experiences.

Practice learning is a valuable experience that needs preparation and active involvement in order for you to develop and demonstrate professional practice competence. They are also crucial for your future employability, that is, the likelihood of you getting a job when you qualify. Drawing on knowledge of the healthcare field, teaching and social work, this chapter begins with an introduction to professional standards and notions of competence. It then considers the basis for ethical decision-making in practice and the approaches that are valued by service users and patients. The skills that accompany ethical practice and a service user or patient-centred approach are also those that enhance your employability. The chapter concludes with an opportunity to consider your learning needs prior to a practice learning context and highlights an approach to help you develop your practice learning agreement.

Key concepts

National occupational standards

Throughout public service work in the UK there are a range of agencies whose role is to ensure that there are enough professionals in place to meet the country's needs, for example, for nurses, social workers or teachers. Known as Public Statutory Regulatory Bodies (PSRBs), they define the required standards for practice and regulate practitioners through professional registration and requirements for continuing professional development. National occupational standards are those statements of the knowledge, values and skills against which you are assessed in learning and in practice and which form the basis of quality in practice.

Competence and fitness to practise

Competence is your attainment when assessed against the national occupational standards. These standards are usually assessed through a combination of written work, for example, an essay reflecting on your practice in a particular situation, and observation of your practice by a mentor or similarly qualified professional. Many programmes require you to produce a portfolio of evidence of your competence for assessment. Competence is closely associated with notions of 'fitness for practice' or 'fitness to practise'. These terms are sometimes used interchangeably; however they do refer to different things – 'fitness for practice' is an assessment of your competence prior to undertaking a practice learning placement. You may undertake a test in your first year to determine if it is safe for you to work with members of the public. Where you undertake and pass a practice learning placement this will count as an assessment of your 'fitness for practice' for your next placement. 'Fitness to practise' is the responsibility of your college or university, your practice learning provider and the PSRB. This is because 'fitness to practise' can concern issues of incompetence, poor practice or bringing the profession into disrepute. A 'fitness to practise' concern can lead to a disciplinary hearing and removal from the professional register of qualified practitioners.

Ethical and moral decision-making

Ethics, values and morals pervade work with people in need. PSRBs and membership organisations such as the health colleges and the College of Social Work produce codes of practice, values statements or codes of ethics that encapsulate the approaches and behaviour expected of a moral practitioner. Codes of practice and codes of ethics are different in that the former focus on the outcomes and actions of the practitioner, whereas the latter also frame the thinking and processes of the practitioner in reaching a particular decision. In focusing on actions codes of practice can inadvertently create a divide between theory and practice; codes of ethics highlight the principles and beliefs necessary for practice. It is important that you understand the context of the various codes that inform practice and the effect that these may have on professional behaviour.

Employability

The Enhancing Student Employability Co-Ordination Team defines employability as:

> *a set of achievements – skills, understandings and personal attributes – that make graduates more likely to gain employment and be successful in their chosen occupations, which benefits themselves, the workforce, the community and the economy.*

(Yorke, 2004, p8)

Employability is not the same as employment, since economic and other circumstances determine the availability of jobs at any one time. However, developing your employability can make employment more likely. This is because notions of employability extend narrow definitions of competence beyond professionally deterministic concepts of knowledge, skills and values to include achievements and attributes that exist beyond professional boundaries. So assessment of professional competence will depend on evidence of intervention based on your knowledge of the law, policy and critical application of techniques or models and methods of intervention. Prospective employers want this too but they also require evidence of softer skills such as the ability to communicate with service users or patients since you need to be able to empathise, be humble and able to empower service users or patients as experts in their own care. Such attributes also extend to good practice with other professionals and include evidence of good team-working skills, good time-keeping and working with integrity.

Professional bodies

There are three main types of body or organisation that have an impact on professional practice. These are PSRBs, professional bodies and trade unions. In the health sector in particular, the professional bodies, usually professional colleges such as the British Association of Occupational Therapists/College of Occupational Therapists, may have a dual role as professional body and trade union.

A number of PSRBs govern work with people in the UK. PSRBs are at arm's length from the government but they fulfil a statutory role in the regulation of practice and professionals and they are mandated by legislation. The main PSRBs are the Health Professions Council, which regulates 16 professions, including social work; the Nursing and Midwifery Council, which, as its name suggests, is responsible for nurses and midwives; and the Teaching Agency, which is an executive agency of the Department for Education, with responsibility for teaching and early-years work. There is no PSRB as defined here for youth and community work, although similar functions are fulfilled by the National Youth Agency, a charity working in partnership with government. The devolved administrations in Northern Ireland, Scotland and Wales may also have their own PSRBs.

Each PSRB manages a register of qualified practitioners; indeed, some PSRBs also require students to register as a student professional. Your name must be included on this register for you to work in your chosen profession. The Care Standards Act 2000, for example, established 'social work' as a restricted title profession, meaning that only those who undertake and pass a recognised programme of study and who register with the regulatory body are entitled to call themselves 'social workers'. Penalties including fines and imprisonment are liable if these conditions are not met.

Some roles are not restricted and do not require your name to appear on a register. Nursery or early-years workers, for example, have no registration requirement, although the provision of services is subject to inspection by the Office for Standards in Education, Children's Services and Skills. Leaders and managers in these services are also expected to follow a programme of study in recognition of their responsibilities and, as stated above, issues of quality, standards and qualifications are determined by the Teaching Agency.

As well as national occupational standards, PSRBs may publish a code of conduct or practice that details the professional behaviour expected of those whose names appear on the register. Where the PSRB does not publish a code of conduct this is likely to be maintained by the second type of organisation, the professional body.

ACTIVITY 5.1

All the information you require for this activity is easily available online.

- Identify the relevant PSRB for your chosen profession and access its website. (A good introductory text will be available by opening the 'who we are' or 'what we do' tab.)
- Next, find the section on national occupational standards. (You will need to spend some time perusing the comprehensive lists of knowledge, values and skills.)
- Make a note of the headline standards rather than each individual requirement – you will need these later.
- Use your search skills to find the code of conduct (or ethics) and note the behaviour expected of you both as a student of your profession and later as a qualified professional.

Like PSRBs, professional bodies are concerned with ensuring quality practice and good outcomes for service users and patients. They achieve this by being a voice for the organisation's membership in balancing practitioners' notions of good practice with regulatory ideas of the same. As a result, definitions of good practice tend to be wider and more inclusive than those promoted by PSRBs. These organisations, such as the Royal College of Nursing and the College of Social Work, are developed, managed and led by practitioners and they seek to influence legislation and policy, and therefore the work of PSRBs through lobbying and the dissemination of examples of good practice. They promote the work and integrity of the profession both nationally and internationally and they have a key role in acknowledging and celebrating the successes of individual practitioners and the profession. Many professional bodies also maintain a register of qualified practitioners.

All professional bodies share a common aim in the continuing education and professional development of the profession and accordingly provide members with a number of benefits such as online access to learning materials, a professional library and a peer-reviewed journal containing topical and leading research. These tools are invaluable in your studies and in developing your career. The articles and research available in the library and covered in the journal will provide a contemporary context for your critical analysis and evaluation of your practice.

Trade unions can also be a good source for continuing professional development and many provide courses in negotiation, leadership and representing the interests of others. Whilst they may not publish a peer-reviewed journal of up-to-date research, they are effective in representing your interests in employment matters, including pay and conditions. Where the professional body also acts as a trade union, the different functions of the organisation are clearly delineated (Table 5.1).

ORGANISATION	PRINCIPLES AND ETHICS	POLICIES AND GUIDANCE ON CPD	RESOURCES AVAILABLE	APPLICATION TO MY LEARNING AND CPD
e.g. College of Social Work/ Royal College of Nursing/College of Occupational Therapists	Code of ethics	Note the aims and objectives in supporting and enhancing CPD	e.g. online library, search engine, seminars, peer-reviewed journal, access to communities of interest	The search engine will provide access to research on practice issues. The journal will enhance critical analysis of my practice
Trade union	Duty of care handbook	Note the aims and objectives in supporting and enhancing CPD	e.g. training courses, seminars, published reports	Training course on equality will enhance my knowledge for inclusive practice. Reports will provide a critique of government policy

Table 5.1 **Professional bodies: principles, policies and professional development**
CPD, continuing professional development.

ACTIVITY 5.2
Create a simple grid on a piece of A4 paper, similar to the one in Table 5.1.

- Where the professional body has both an educational and trade union function, consider each role separately.

Comment

In undertaking Activities 5.1 and 5.2 you have developed your knowledge of the requirements, policies and resources pertinent to practice, continuing education and professional development. You will notice that there are many similarities in the aims of PSRBs, professional bodies and trade unions; however there are key differences. PSRBs tend to produce national occupational standards and notions of competence based upon observable or measurable behaviour, such as your ability to complete an assessment or intervention using the requisite tools and forms. They conceptualise competence on the basis of outcomes; that is, on your ability to complete a job well. Professional bodies acknowledge the need for the rules and regulations that govern practice but they also crucially look beyond outcomes to consider the essential qualities and attributes of the practitioner that are necessary to achieve good outcomes.

Thinking about ethical behaviour

The primary determinants of professional behaviour are discussed in depth by Oko (2011), who points out there is an inherent tension in only practising on the basis of the knowledge, values and skills determined by PSRBs. Since PSRBs promote what is measurable or observable, good practice becomes defined by adherence to policy and procedure and the achievement of outcomes. In other words, emphasis is placed upon the act of doing without necessarily including the act of thinking or acting upon the principled beliefs that give each profession its own unique identity. Further understanding of this tension can be developed through investigating the difference between the terms 'ethics', 'moral' and 'values'.

ACTIVITY 5.3
Without reference to the internet, books or other sources, write a definition of the three key terms: 'ethics', 'morals' and 'values'. Now look at how the professional literature defines these terms. It is important to use professional sources, whether print- or web-based, to ensure the accuracy of definition for your profession.

Consider the differences between your own definition and those of the profession as well as differences in meaning of the words.

Comment

'Ethics' refers to the principles and beliefs that define moral behaviour. In other words, ethics is a way of thinking about what is right or wrong in practice. 'Morals' are the rules or codes of behaviour to which society or groups in society, including professional groups, conform. A doctor will understand that murder is wrong but behaves morally when treating the murderer as any other patient. Similarly, a social worker does not condone child abuse when working with a perpetrator. 'Values' refer to the professional and personal beliefs and experiences that influence our thoughts and actions. Influences on your values include family, community, culture and religious beliefs.

Ethical theories and decision-making

Ethics, morals and values, as well as professional knowledge, are key components in decision-making in practice and by now you have realised that there are tensions in their definition and application. PSRBs can present ethical and moral practice as based on rules whereas you and your professional body may expand upon this to include the virtues that you bring to a situation. Banks and Gallagher (2008) explore the potential for tension between four main ethical approaches.

The first approach is based on the work of the eighteenth-century German philosopher, Immanuel Kant, who emphasises respect for rules and the individual patient or service user. The second approach conversely promotes the principles of utility and justice, that is, it is ethical and just to meet the needs of the many rather than the individual. The third approach combines the first two into what has become known as a common morality approach. It is particularly prevalent in medicine and healthcare through the work of Beauchamp and Childress (1994), who promote the principles of autonomy, beneficence, non-maleficence and justice.

These three approaches encourage adherence to rules and duties and, unsurprisingly, they are the backbone of PSRB codes of practice. They also focus on the outcome of an action in following the rules and duties of the profession. However they do not account for the thoughts and virtues of practitioners in applying the rules and undertaking their duties, that is, the motive of practitioners in undertaking a particular action. The importance of considering the motive of the practitioner is alluded to by Howarth (2010):

> If we are really going to achieve child-focused assessments, it is necessary not only to 'see' the child, but also to 'see' the practitioner. Just as for the child this means understanding the child's lived experience and consulting with the child to identify ways of improving life in order to ensure that their needs are met, the same is true for practitioners.
>
> (Howarth, 2010, p14)

The need for you to be reflective and reflexive in your practice is covered in the next chapter. What is also emphasised is the importance of combining the strengths of each of the three previous ethical approaches with a fourth – virtue ethics. Virtue ethics emphasises the intention of the practitioner in undertaking an action rather than just the outcome of that action. The practitioner is an active participant in moral action rather than a passive observer of rules and duties. Virtue approaches necessarily require you to consider the impact of self on a situation in addition to the impact of rules and duties.

How you interpret and act upon the rules and duties of the profession is an important aspect of practice as you will often be in a position of responsibility or power in relation to the patient or service user. For these reasons it is important that you consider all of the influences on your decision-making. Rothman (1998, pp4–22) helpfully identifies four components of ethical decision-making:

1. defining the ethical problem;
2. gathering information relevant to the problem;
3. an appropriate theoretical base must be determined, then professional values explored, service user or patient values understood and the impact of personal values recognised;
4. options must be weighed and a sound decision reached.

> **ACTIVITY 5.4**
> Revisit the codes of ethics or codes of practice promoted by your relevant PSRB and professional body. Read the following case study and decide what you would do based on the PSRB codes, the professional body codes and your personal value base. Use Rothman's four components to guide you.

CASE STUDY 5.1

You are working for a childcare organisation that has an unbreakable rule that states 'under no circumstances should a member of staff have physical contact with a child or young person'. There are several reasons for this, including protecting the child, protecting you and protecting the integrity of the organisation and the childcare profession. You are working with a group of children outside one day and you hear a commotion; a five year old girl approaches you crying and in obvious distress although there are no obvious injuries. As she reaches you she raises her arms to be lifted up. What do you do?

Comment

This scenario provides an interesting ethical dilemma, the type of which is an everyday occurrence in practice. If you lift the child and break the rules then you may be held to be in breach of policy and procedure and not yet competent according to PSRB requirements. If you don't lift the child you may conversely contravene a primary goal of the profession, for example, compassion and putting the needs of service users or patients first. So, what do you do?

If you straightforwardly say that you would not lift the child since you cannot break the rule, you cannot be held to be wrong since you have made a moral decision; your argument would be that you considered and followed the rule. However, has such a decision been made by thinking about and evaluating all of the information available to you, including your personal value base, the impact of self on the situation and the type of person you want to be?

In Chapter 1 we asked you to think about your understanding of and approach to learning and pointed out the differences between surface and deep approaches to learning. A surface learner will only be concerned with meeting the requirements as set out by the PSRB; a deep learner will be similarly concerned but will also explicitly understand the process of decision-making that led to a moral decision. A deep learner will show consideration of the rules but will also demonstrate that the process of decision-making included understanding of and adherence to the ethics and morals of the profession and consideration of the impact of self. In the scenario there is no right or wrong answer; however, there is a defensible and moral answer. Preparation for practice involves critical understanding of the rules and regulations that govern the profession and, since no set of rules or regulations can cover every possible dilemma that might present (Banks and Gallagher, 2008), it also requires explicit exposure of the personal values and experiences through which moral decisions are made. In particular, if you decide to lift the child, what were your motives?

Developing as an ethical and employable practitioner

The ethical practitioner is someone who is able to balance a range of competing demands, including the rules of the profession, with the moral foundations of the profession and personal values. Ethical and moral practice is at the heart of practice learning and the ethical and moral practitioner is one who works in partnership with service users or patients and who seeks to empower them to take as much responsibility as is permissible for their own care. Service users have identified the conditions under which they feel empowered when working in partnership with practitioners involved in their care:

- when honesty and trust has been developed;
- through open and clear communication;
- through genuine involvement in the process;
- when empathy and genuine concern are evident;
- when practice is accountable – enabling the service user to challenge what is said and written (Millar and Corby, 2006, pp887–899).

Such an approach requires effective communication and other 'soft skills' which are equally prized by employers.

Honesty and trust are based on a number of things, including your knowledge of your own and others' strengths and those aspects of your knowledge, skills and values that require enhancement. They require you to be reflective and reflexive, to consider the impact of self, and to recognise what you don't know as well as what you do know. This includes the ability to be humble, to accept responsibility for tasks and to act on your initiative as a member of a larger team.

Good communication is also key to honesty and integrity. This involves the ability to communicate effectively in written form and in person. For the latter, the ability to recognise and respond to another person's body language and to use emotional intelligence is important. Presenting, listening, willingness and skills in giving and receiving constructive criticism are also important components of good communication.

Genuine involvement in the process includes encouraging and empowering service users or patients to make decisions on their own behalf as far as circumstances allow. Influencing, motivating, negotiating, summarising and persuading are all elements that support genuine involvement, as are your ability to undertake tasks and to complete them on time. Your willingness to turn up for an appointment on time and your capacity to evaluate with the service user or patient and to make the necessary changes are also crucial.

Empathy requires you to understand the situation from the other person's point of view; this is not the same as to sympathise but instead refers to the ability to show understanding and concern for that person's situation. You should be able to collect, collate, synthesise and assess information from a situation in an organised and timely fashion. Being empathic may also require lateral thinking and openness to new situations and new learning through reflection in action.

Being accountable involves indepth knowledge of the law, policies, procedures, theories and methods relevant to another person's life. In addition you need to be able to plan effectively, work to deadlines and prioritise in stressful and conflicting situations. The overall aim is attention to quality. Remember too that accountability involves adherence to rules and professional duties as well as accountability to the service user or patient through critical self-reflection of the impact of personal values and experience.

Table 5.2 provides an overview of the skills and attributes that are essential to developing partnership with service users and patients and for employability. The attributes are indicative rather than inclusive and you should seek to expand them as you continue your studies.

> ### ACTIVITY 5.5
> Consider your current skills relating to partnership working and employability by completing a SWOT analysis of your skills.

SWOT is an acronym for strengths, weaknesses, opportunities and threats. For this activity refer to the skills and attributes in Table 5.2 and undertake a self-assessment of your current attainment against them. Strengths refer to those skills for which you have already demonstrated competence. Try to give explicit evidence of your strengths in particular. Weaknesses are those skills that require enhancement. Opportunities are those situations and people that will enable you to enhance your skills. Threats are those situations and people that may impede your learning and development. Table 5.3 will help.

Comment

It is important that you include those skills and attributes you have identified as weaknesses for enhancement within your practice learning agreement and discuss them openly with your mentor or practice teacher from the outset.

You may notice that strengths and weaknesses concentrate on a range of issues internal to you, including your personal motivation, skills, feelings and values. Opportunities and threats concentrate on the range of external issues that can affect your studies and practice, including expertise of others, career demands and problems that may arise in university or at home.

Preparing for placement

In completing the SWOT analysis you are beginning to prepare for placement and to be explicit about your learning needs. It is also helpful to think about some of the people and processes that will help your learning and development.

Practice learning mentor/practice teacher

You will have a named mentor or practice teacher who will play a key role in your learning. In addition to supporting you and managing your work on a day-to-day basis your mentor or practice teacher provides models of good practice and helps you to develop as a reflective practitioner. You should recognise the contribution made by mentors or practice teachers to your learning and appreciate their generosity in giving their time to help you to learn. Ultimately

ATTRIBUTES FOR EMPOWERMENT AND PARTNERSHIP WORKING (MILLAR AND CORBY, 2006)	SKILLS FOR EMPLOYABILITY	
	CATEGORIES	ATTRIBUTES
Honesty and trust	Professionalism in managing work, learning and continuing professional development	Reflection and reflexiveness, including knowledge of impact of self Learning Humility Quality focus Use of initiative and willingness to accept tasks
Open and clear communication	Communicating	Written Face to face Listening Presenting Willingness and skills in giving and receiving constructive criticism
Genuine involvement in the process	Social interaction, maintenance and development	Time management Influencing Motivating Negotiating Summarising Openness to new situatlons and new learning through reflection in action Evaluating
Empathy and genuine concern	Problem-solving	Communication Lateral thinking Information retrieval and assessment Analysing Co-operating
Accountable practice	Team working	Plan effectively Work to deadlines Prioritise Team working Accept and use constructive criticism Information retrieval and handling

Table 5.2 **Employability skills – an indicative rather than inclusive list of attributes**

STRENGTHS	WEAKNESSES
Written and face-to-face communication – evidence by feedback from service users/patients and colleagues, including line manager Team working – good relationships with peers, can complete tasks on time, can give and take instructions	Time keeping – leave some tasks to the last minute and find it difficult to fit everything into my week Don't always prioritise
OPPORTUNITIES	THREATS
Tutor and mentor/practice teacher can help Time management tools available Use a diary	Competing demands from family and friends when busy Like socialising Can't say no!

Table 5.3 **SWOT analysis**

mentors and practice teachers help to assess the quality of your practice. This is an important role and where possible mentors and practice teachers will:

- have experience of acting as a mentor, practice teacher or supervisor;
- hold a recognised professional qualification relevant to context;
- be registered with the relevant professional body for their profession;
- have been qualified for a minimum period of time, for example, two years.

The learning agreement

The learning agreement is the starting point for all practice learning. It establishes a set of agreed learning needs for you which can then be discussed throughout the placement. Achievements and problems can be identified. A form is usually provided and must be completed by you together with your mentor or practice teacher at the beginning of each practice learning placement. The SWOT analysis will help you to identify your learning needs. This is a working document and should be revisited periodically during your practice learning.

Ongoing consultation or supervision

You can expect that informal consultation or supervision will be ongoing; however there will also be opportunities for discussion that are formal and developmental. It is assumed that the mentor or practice teacher will have the experience and skills to take on the task and it is vital that both you and she prepare for consultation/supervision. An agenda should be agreed with notes taken and a copy kept by both parties. Do not assume that it is solely the mentor's or practice teacher's responsibility to take the notes.

There is likely to be a form for you to record consultation/supervision. These records are formative and are helpful when reflecting on your development.

The tutor

You will be assigned a tutor who is responsible for supporting you through the programme. The tutor will be expected to:

- ensure completion of a learning agreement in consultation with you and the mentor/practice teacher and to ensure that the agreement is updated as necessary;
- support and advise you in the preparation of your assessments;
- hold tutorials with you to discuss your written work and generally to promote your progression through practice learning;
- participate in meetings with you and your mentor or practice teacher as necessary;
- assess, in conjunction with the mentor and practice teacher, your written work.

You

You have clear roles and responsibilities and must treat practice learning as if it were a paid job. Good time management, punctuality, reliability and commitment are vital. You must meet the requirements of placement as if you were an employee.

Your role is to be proactive in negotiating your own learning needs with the tutor and mentor/ practice teacher, in order to demonstrate an appropriate level of self-reliance in professional and academic competence. You will develop a learning agreement and will undertake to work in negotiation with the mentor/practice teacher and to co-operate with the requirements in providing evidence of your practice. You will be available to attend meetings and tutorials and will prepare practice evidence in line with the requirements and guidance for your programme of study.

When you are undertaking practice learning you need to realise that you are operating in a professional capacity rather than as a student. Being a professional worker brings with it a range of responsibilities and means that you have to be aware of the standards of professional conduct which are required. You should be aware of the following issues:

- care and responsibility: as workers, you have a responsibility to act in the best interest of the children, young people and adults with whom you are working;
- non-discriminatory behaviour: you must act in a non-discriminatory way at all times and adhere to the spirit and the letter of the practice learning agency's equal opportunities policies;
- confidentiality: you should respect the confidences you receive. If you wish to use or discuss situations containing personal or confidential information during your studies, for example in assessed work to demonstrate competence, the information should be presented so as to ensure the anonymity of everyone involved.

Reflective recordings or diary

It is recommended that you make reflective recordings on a regular basis and they should be more than just a description of the activities you have been involved in on a particular day. You are expected to think, for example, about the theories, values and skills used and to reflect upon the success of the activity (or not). Reflection on practice is an integral part of your learning and is covered in more detail in the next chapter.

REFLECTION POINT

In Activity 5.1 you identified the national occupational standards for your chosen profession. Revisit these – it will be easier to consider the headline categories rather than the individual statements of competence.

- Complete a SWOT analysis of your current attainment against the standards. Where you have identified areas for enhancement, include these on your learning agreement.

CHAPTER SUMMARY

- Completion of the activities in this chapter will help you to prepare for practice learning and to have explicit ideas about your learning needs and ethical practice.
- Practice learning is more than just work experience – it is an opportunity to demonstrate your competence against the required national occupational standards of your profession and also involves your continuing professional development.
- Reflection and reflexiveness are important skills. You need to consider the impact of self when working with those in need and to think about those virtues that make a good worker. Such an approach is also indicative of an ethical and moral practitioner. You will find that the skills that enable partnership with and empowerment of service users or patients are also prized by employers.
- It is important that you prepare for practice learning by undertaking a self-assessment of your current knowledge, values and skills and incorporate areas for enhancement with your learning agreement; practice is, over all, about learning.

The final chapter turns to the importance of reflection as an aid to learning and the importance of becoming a reflective practitioner.

FURTHER READING

Doel, M and Shardlow, M (2009) *Educating Professionals: Practice learning in health and social care.* Farnham: Ashgate.

This book uses case examples from nine professions to explore roles, areas of expertise and general concepts across professions. The authors focus on student learning in practice settings: how this is organised, what methods are used and how abilities are assessed.

Parker, J (2004) *Effective Practice Learning in Social Work.* Exeter: Learning Matters.

A useful and accessible book for students from a range of professional programmes. This book explains how experience can deliver a unique learning opportunity for students and is ideal for those about to undertake a placement.

6 UNDERSTANDING AND USING REFLECTION

CHAPTER OBJECTIVES

By the end of this chapter you should be able to:

- define what is meant by reflection and comprehend that it is an aid to developing understanding and enhancing your learning;

- recognise the importance of reflecting on your placement experiences in order to make links between theory and practice;

- identify a range of models that can be used for developing and demonstrating reflection in your written work.

Introduction

The concept of reflection is central to the education of many professionals, including, of course, those working within health and social care and educational settings. As part of your formal learning, you will be expected to develop and demonstrate this skill in your academic work as well as showing evidence of reflecting on your practice experiences.

In this chapter we will look at what is meant by the term 'reflection' as well as some of its derivatives, such as 'reflexivity' and 'critical reflection'. We also demonstrate how you are expected to show your understanding of your subject matter as a 'reflective practitioner', through your professional values, skills and knowledge and as part of your academic and professional development.

Defining reflection

Reflection is a structured approach to thinking that looks back on an experience or event that has occurred. It is a cognitive activity that involves the mental process of selection, attention and analysis in order to develop or deepen our understanding of something and enhance our capacity to know or do something (action) differently in the future. In this respect, reflection transforms an experience into knowledge (Knott and Scragg, 2007, p6).

Unpicking this definition, we can begin to see some key characteristics of the reflective process.

- It is a purposeful approach to thinking back about something – be it an incident or event or an experience (selection).
- It involves an examination of the material from different angles or perspectives and acts as an interrogative process that examines the event in more detail (attention).
- It seeks out meaning (analysis) in order to develop and enhance understanding and uses this understanding or insight to know or do things differently in the future (action).

Reflecting on your learning experiences, whether these arise from the classroom or from practice experiences, is a key part of developing your understanding of your subject area with subsequent use of this new knowledge so that you can develop in your professional role.

In Chapter 1, we looked at definitions of learning and invited you to come up with a definition of learning.

ACTIVITY 6.1
Look back to Activity 1.1 and revise your understanding of what learning means based upon our definition.

We suggested that learning involves a cognitive process of active engagement with the new learning material in order to promote meaning-making and understanding. We also made the distinction between deep and surface approaches to learning. Deep learning is likely to lead to greater long-term retention of new information, since we use this information to build on what we already know and ask how this new material enables us to make better sense or give us a more all-round conception of the subject.

In contrast, a surface or superficial approach to learning sees learning as a disparate or random collection of information that is more likely to encourage memorisation of key facts, but it remains disconnected and does not link to previous knowledge and does not promote the process of meaning-making and building understanding.

Being reflective is a key part of developing a deep approach to learning, but while this approach to learning seeks to build up a picture, reflection takes a small part of the picture (i.e. selection) and subjects it to exploration and interrogation (attention) and considers new interpretations and understanding (analysis). When we reflect, whether as a result of our learning experiences in the classroom or placement experiences, we are effectively examining an aspect of this learning experience in order to enhance our understanding. The aim is new knowledge so that we can do things better in the future. For Bolton (2005) reflective practice (that is, the act of being reflective) is learning and developing through examining what we think happened on any occasion and, at its simplest, suggests that reflection can be a means of *practical problem-solving: asking ourselves:*

- *what happened?*
- *why?*
- *what do I think and feel about it?*
- *how can I do it better next time?*

(Bolton, 2005, p9)

We can see why reflection is described as an interrogative process which involves the re-examination of an event or experience – we go back over something, examining it in more detail, in order to develop a clearer understanding. However, seeing reflection just as a means of problem-solving can suggest that the reflector remains unchanged by the experience. A more sophisticated appreciation of reflection sees the spotlight of analysis fall on the reflector as well, acknowledging that you are changed and influenced by your experiences as you reflect back on them. With the spotlight of analysis on you, you should also ask yourself:

- how does this re-examination of a particular event enhance your understanding of yourself?

And, as a means of learning from your experience:

- how can you use this understanding or insight of yourself to improve an aspect of your development as a beginning student or practitioner?

Continuing with building up a definition, we can add three more features that characterise reflection:

1. It is a contemplative process, as suggested by terms such as 'interrogative' and 'examination' – we need time to select an event and subject it to the reflective process.
2. In beginning to analyse and make sense of the experience, it is also a means of focusing back on one's self – you also become the object of analysis. It is not just trying to make sense of something, as a kind of neutral observer so to speak, but it is a close examination of your actions and feelings in the event as well.
3. Recognition of our feelings or emotions is a key part of the reflective process.

This last point is important because it sees reflection as moving towards a deeper level of analysis with ourselves at the heart of that analysis. We re-examine our motives, our feelings, our behaviour and the consequences of our actions as part of trying to gain a deeper understanding of the situation and ourselves in that situation. This is suggestive of the term 'reflexivity'.

Reflexivity and critical reflection

Bolton (2005) describes this deeper level of reflection as 'reflexivity' – it is a means of *making aspects of the self strange: focusing close attention upon one's own actions, thoughts, feelings, values, identity and their effect upon others, situation and professional and social structures* (p10). Being reflexive means that we are not just observers of social situations, but acknowledges that we are also part of that situation – we are both products and creators of our social world. However, rather than interpreting and making sense of things only from our own point of view, in making aspects of ourselves strange, we re-examine our behaviour, thoughts and motives and recognise how these factors shape and influence how we see and make sense of things. In turn, we see how others may see and experience us as well. We recognise there are alternative explanations about ourselves. By adopting a deeper analysis of ourselves, we can use these new insights and understandings for the benefit of developing ourselves more fully, essential for a student and a beginning practitioner. As Sheppard (2007) observes, *the reflexive practitioner shows a high degree of self-awareness, role awareness and awareness of assumptions underlying their practice* (p129). This *high degree of awareness of assumptions underpinning your practice* marks out another dimension of the reflexive process, which is often described as 'critical reflection'.

For learning purposes, however, it is important to realise that the word 'critical' is not used in its everyday sense – it is not about being negative and making negative comments about one's own or others' beliefs or actions. Instead, critical thinking skills are fundamental to developing a deep approach to learning and an understanding of your subject area. For academic purposes, being critical refers to an ability to analyse both positive and negative features of something; to consider both the strengths and weaknesses of the case and to be able to evaluate what worked well as well as what did not work well. As Cottrell (2011) states: *Good critical analysis accounts for why something is good or poor, why it works or fails. It is not enough to merely list good and bad points* (p8).

Summarising the components of critical reflection, it involves:

- critically analysing and evaluating an aspect of our professional practice, academic learning or a significant event/experience;
- gaining new understandings and appreciations of the way we think and behave by examining the event from different perspectives and different levels of detail;
- an awareness of our self and exploring the feelings and emotions associated with the situation;
- a consideration of external sources of authority or knowledge, i.e. research, theory, professional knowledge to help us evaluate or judge our experiences;
- an attempt to make sense and develop a deeper understanding of the event you are examining;
- using your new understanding to effect change, both in yourself and for the benefit of others in your professional role.

(adapted from Brown and Rutter, 2006, p17 and Cottrell, 2011, pp208–209)

As you can see, in developing a comprehensive understanding of the reflective process, it is important that you realise that reflection is more than simply looking back and attempting to problem-solve or question an event. Rather than making a distinction between reflection, reflexivity and critical reflection, in this book we have combined the three terms and refer to deep or critical reflection as incorporating all these definitions. Being critically reflective involves an examination of yourself and your feelings and motives and how these feelings shape your understanding of the event. In turn, you arrive at recognition that you also shape the event under examination as well.

Being a critically reflective student means that you subject your analysis of the event to external sources of authority; that is, you draw upon the established knowledge sources of your subject area so that you are able to make an informed judgment about your understanding of the event to justify your reasoning. You begin to make links between your reflective experiences and the established theory of your subject area.

This deeper level of reflection can make learning a *transformative process* (Mezirow, 1991), whereby learners are introduced to *new ways of talking, thinking and knowing* [and those that] *critically reflect upon their beliefs and assumptions frequently come to challenge taken-for-granted social practices, ideologies and norms* (Miller and Sambell, 2003, pp8–9).

Cottrell (2011) concludes:

a key aim of critical reflection is to transform the way you see the world, or an aspect of it, such that you think and act differently. . . [at its best] *reflection can have a transformative quality, with a profound effect on your being and sense of self, others and the world around you.*

(Cottrell, 2011, p209)

REFLECTION POINT

Take a few minutes to think about what you have just read and come up with a definition of reflection.

Being reflective is a contemplative process – it takes time to think about an event and subject it to the reflective process. So it is not possible to be reflective all of the time. Instead, reflection is most likely to involve thinking about a significant event that has had an impact on you and your definition should include some of the following key points.

- It is a structured approach to thinking about a significant event and involves examining and interrogating the experience from different angles or perspectives.
- As a means of enhancing our understanding, reflection is an aid to learning and self-development, making sense of ourselves, our practice experiences and our classroom experiences.
- In attempting to enhance our understanding, we should draw upon established and up-to-date knowledge sources of our subject area, including research, theory and practice learning experiences so that we are not just relying on our own interpretation of events.

Why is reflection important?

Reflection is a key part of developing a deep approach to learning. It is a means of helping you make sense and so enhance your understanding. You are using your previous knowledge and understanding of the subject to help you make sense of the new material of learning, effectively relating the new material to what you already know. In this way, you are piecing the new learning material together in order to develop a more coherent understanding of your discipline. Moon (1999) refers to this level of learning as meaning-making, where we draw upon a range of knowledge sources to integrate what we know and what we are trying to understand in order to enhance or improve our learning. New learning becomes meaningful either because it is linked to what the learner already knows – in everyday language, we are able to take on board this new material of learning – or else we have to make more of an effort to process or accommodate this new learning and fit it together with what we already know so that our understanding is enhanced – we build upon and build up our understanding (Moon, 1999, pp108–111).

In the classroom setting, good teaching and learning strategies will be used to support you in the process of meaning-making. Peer group learning, that is, working in small groups with others in your class on a particular learning activity, is an effective way of helping to develop your understanding and consolidate your learning. So, for instance, you might be asked to work on a case study, where the main aim of the learning task is to help you make links with what you have just been learning about and how this can make sense or fits into a practice context. You may be studying an aspect of social policy in relation to young people and homelessness and are then given a case study in which you are asked to make decisions about eligibility criteria which can lead you to begin to critique the concept of 'homelessness' and 'need'. In doing so, you come to realise that such terms are not as straightforward or uncontroversial as they may have first seemed.

You may be asked to watch a DVD of, or visit, preschool children in an early-years setting with the aim of helping to develop your understanding of an aspect of child development. Again, you may come to develop a more critical understanding of this area and see that not all children conform to textbook explanations of how children behave at a particular age or stage of development. Other innovative learning activities may include the use of photographic images which can help you critique taken-for-granted ideas and beliefs, say around disability. The photographs act as prompts to promote discussion and help reveal common ideas and assumptions that can be held about people with a disability. Drawing on your formal classroom learning, this can be used as a means of developing alternative explanations that move away from an individual focus on the disability to one that emphasises the importance of antidiscriminatory practice theory and the social model of disability and so help to highlight the role that (able-bodied) society plays in 'dis-abling' people with impairments and excluding them from full social and economic inclusion in our society (Thompson, 2006).

Working in a small group is an effective way of promoting learning since, with the support of your teacher, you are encouraged to participate in discussions around the learning task, sharing your ideas and understanding. In this way, group work can encourage students to take responsibility for their learning and help develop self-confidence and interpersonal communication skills. Group work is a collaborative process and can help foster group cohesion, helping you to feel a part of the learning environment as well. When well-managed, group work encourages you to engage more fully with the content of the subject; it is an effective learning strategy for encouraging a deep approach to learning (Griffiths, 1999).

ACTIVITY 6.2

Drawing on your understanding of the reflective process, write a short account (no longer than one side of A4 paper) of your experience of a learning activity that you have undertaken, e.g. a case study or a discussion group, focusing on what was most significant in terms of helping you to make better sense of your new learning.

Comment

Hopefully, you are able to identify an aspect of your learning experience that was significant and helped to develop your understanding. Later in this chapter, we will look at models of reflection that you can use to help develop your reflective writing style. In relation to helping you develop a more holistic understanding of your subject area, remember that group seminars or individual tutorials with the module leader also serve the same purpose – they are designed to help encourage a guided discussion of the subject matter and encourage understanding. You should also remember that good teachers provide ongoing feedback throughout your lessons as you progress through each module and that feedback is not just confined to individual feedback on an assessed piece of work.

The reflective practitioner

The term 'reflective practitioner' is used specifically to refer to you demonstrating your learning about professional practice during your placements in health, social welfare or educational settings. To be reflective in your placement settings is about how you demonstrate your learning from this experience – it transforms an experience into knowledge because your experience has been of benefit to you and as a result you can show evidence of learning from it. So the same skills of critical reflection are still necessary on placement: you are expected to interrogate and analyse significant events that have had an impact on you, thinking about how you feel about it and what you did and drawing on your formal knowledge sources to help develop a richer understanding and inform your practice.

Cottrell (2011, p225) identifies four important reasons for critically reflecting on your placement experiences.

1. It anchors theory in meaningful, concrete experience, helping to bring it alive.

Case Study 6.1

Alison is in her first year on an Early Childhood Studies degree. She undertook a three-day observational placement in a nursery and was asked to keep a reflective account of her learning experiences. One of the things that struck Alison as significant was the use of behavioural methods by the staff to manage the children's behaviour. In particular, Alison was able to make links with her academic learning about behaviourism and the idea of modelling (Bandura, 1977) and social learning theory and how young children might copy an aspect of the staff's behaviour, as well as how the children were influenced by other children's behaviour. She also noted the use of another behaviour technique by staff, based on the work of Skinner (1904–90), where a system of rewards and punishment was used to encourage good behaviour or modify unwanted behaviour in the children.

---

2. It gives recognition to learning gained in non-academic contexts.

The workplace can offer both rich and challenging learning experiences to you as a student on placement. A significant comment that is often made by students is the difference between the high standards of practice that are encouraged in the university and the reality of being in the workplace where students might observe a sharp contrast between classroom theory and the reality of practice. Alternatively, students can learn a lot from observing colleagues and how they might manage a meeting, say with parents, or how to deal with difficult behaviour in a young child, or how to introduce themselves when they have to make a professional phone call. In addition, experienced practitioners can share their 'practice wisdom' with new students, and give them tips, for instance, on how to complete an aspect of some paperwork or useful agencies or people to talk to in the office who might be helpful. Alison from Case study 6.1 might share her experiences of being a novice, helping her to feel less anxious and to 'normalise' her experience of being on placement.

3. It provides a bridge between practical experience and academic study.

CASE STUDY 6.2

Marcus was an experienced youth worker who was undertaking a Youth Studies foundation degree. In his reflective journal he noted how his studies had enabled him to think more critically about his work practices as a youth worker. He felt he was now not 'just doing the job' based upon experience and familiarity with the task, but was increasingly more able to think critically about what he was doing and why, drawing upon the theories and research he had learnt at college. He was feeling increasingly more confident in his ability to explain and justify his practice and interventions with young people based upon his formal learning from class.

4. It helps develop understanding of difficult work situations, improving professional practice.

This last point is suggestive of the fact that practice in the helping professions is not always straightforward or indeed non-controversial. Again, it can challenge what is learnt at college or university when you are faced with conflicting or difficult situations in the workplace. Typical scenarios include: working with other professionals whose role and focus of intervention are different to yours or working with families or individuals who may resent professional intervention or have an unrealistic expectation about what you can do in your professional role. Bear in mind that professional practice can bring us face to face with issues that resonate with our own personal experiences, making the work more challenging or difficult. Such conflicts highlight the importance of professional values and ethics and learning how to resolve these difficulties whilst still promoting good practice and maintaining professional relationships with the people you work with and the people who use the services of your agency.

Reflection in supervision

Learning how to manage effectively difficult or troubling situations in the workplace calls to mind the importance of a secure learning environment and a supportive practice teacher or mentor who can help you disentangle and explore your feelings and thoughts around such issues. Howe (2009) describes this as an important opportunity for *emotional thinking* and represents *good reflective supervision* (pp173–174).

Reflective supervision means that as a student on placement, you have the opportunity to evaluate the whole domain of your practice experiences. This includes the agency you are in, the work of other colleagues and professionals you meet in the course of your placement, others who contribute to the work of the agency, the underpinning knowledge, skills and values of your professional work setting and the formal knowledge that you have learnt as part of your studies, and of course, you will be asked to reflect on your own practice and your contact with the people who use the agency's services. Opening up to scrutiny the whole of your placement learning opportunities can lead to a consideration of different and improved methods of practice as you think critically about the explanations that you draw upon to help you make sense of what you are doing, and explore your thoughts and feelings about yourself as a student on placement who is beginning to take on a professional role. Using supervision is a key opportunity for developing your reflective skills: here you can show evidence of being able to integrate what you learnt in your studies at college and transfer your understanding and knowledge to the workplace. At the same time, the reflective process allows you to think about your practice experiences and how these connect with your classroom learning, and so demonstrate a link between theory and practice.

Writing reflectively

In this final section, we are looking at developing your reflective written skills through the use of different models of reflection. At the beginning of the chapter when we were building up a definition of reflection, one of the things we mentioned was that reflection is a contemplative process – it takes time to order your thoughts and feelings about an event that has had an impact on you. We are not always able to process or make sense of this event immediately in order to present a coherent account. On placement you are expected to prepare and plan for supervision, having some idea of the issues that you want to focus on and clarify.

Equally, in your studies at university, the process of understanding and making sense is not always straightforward either and so, for both settings, it is likely that you will be asked to record your thoughts and feelings about the breadth of your learning experiences in a reflective journal or diary. On the basis of your accounts, you are likely to be required to write up an aspect of your learning experiences for an assessed piece of work – whether it is in relation to your practice learning for inclusion in your practice portfolio or for a specific module taught at university. For both settings, however, remember your practice teacher, mentor or university lecturer will be looking for a theorised piece of writing which shows evidence of learning by being able to make links with the underpinning knowledge, values and skills associated with your subject area and the occupational standards associated with your profession.

ACTIVITY 6.3

Identify a significant event that has had an impact on you. Whether this was on placement or in the classroom, identify key elements that need to be included in a reflective written account.

Comment

Reflective writing should include the following:

- a short, factual description of the event under consideration;
- an exploration of your initial thoughts, feelings and assumptions about the situation;
- a deeper level of analysis that begins to look at the event from different perspectives and considers alternative explanations;
- these alternative explanations should begin to link to some aspect of your formal learning – this is what is meant by theorising. Being reflective, for formal academic purposes, should draw upon the knowledge, skills and values acquired as part of your studies as a means of helping you reach a more developed understanding of the incident.

You should be able to use this revised understanding to enhance your practice or an aspect of your learning.

Although the issues that prompt us to reflect may often be ill defined and, by their nature, difficult to make sense of, you should still remember that reflection is a structured approach to thinking and therefore your writing needs to be structured and follow a coherent pattern in order to demonstrate your thinking process and show an attempt at making sense of the experience.

You must be clear about the purpose for which you are writing. If you are writing for an assessed piece of work, then there will be a specific set of marking criteria, so make sure you understand what is being asked of you and that you understand the criteria that are being used to judge the quality of your work. If you are not sure, then ask the person who is marking the work for more clarity and guidance.

In contrast, you may be asked to write a reflective account of an experience on placement for supervision purposes with your mentor. In this case, the work may not be assessed in the sense that you receive a mark or grade for it, but instead, the purpose of the reflective account is to show your understanding of the issue and for your supervisor to help you in your learning.

Whether the purpose of your writing is for an assessed piece of work, or personal reflections in a journal or diary or for use in supervision, your reflections should lead you to do things differently in the future and show evidence of learning. So, if you have done something well – be it on placement or received a good mark for a piece of assessed work at university – when you reflect upon this, the aim of your reflections is to know how you can reproduce a good piece of work or how you can improve your work for the future. It is not enough to conclude that the work was good or otherwise, but rather, that you are clear about:

- what you did;
- why it was effective or not helpful;
- how you can use this insight in the future to improve your practice and learning.

To develop your reflective writing skills, models of reflection are useful because they provide a framework that helps structure your thinking. They provide prompts for our thinking and help to ensure that we work through the whole of the process of reflection in enough depth to be able to find new insights or understandings that can be applied in the future (Healey and Spencer, 2008).

Models of reflection

Models of reflection can vary in complexity due to the number of stages or prompts that are used to help break down the process of reflection. In essence, however, they contain key features. They ask you to:

- describe;
- analyse;
- action plan for the future.

Staged models

Borton (1970) simplifies the reflective process into three stages:

1. What?
2. So what?
3. Now what?

'What?' refers to the description of the event. The reader needs to know what it is that you are reflecting on, so inevitably you have to give an account of it. The description should be as factual and succinct as possible. It is not a story but an account of what happened and how you felt, so only relevant information needs to be included – there is no attempt to go into detail at this stage. Even so, you still need to think carefully about describing the event for written purposes.

'So what?' prompts the beginning of your analysis: so what is significant about the event you are describing? You are beginning to interrogate and examine in more detail your thoughts and feelings about the event: what did you think or feel? What is the basis for your thoughts or assumptions? Why did you think that or why did something happen? Can you justify or explain these thoughts in more detail? It is not enough to state: *I was anxious* or *It made me angry*. The reader wants to know why you were angry or anxious. In exploring the question 'why?' you examine the experience from different points of views and consider alternative explanations. Maybe you were angry because you were frustrated about somebody's behaviour which you felt was obstructive, but re-examining this from a different perspective other than your own you can begin to appreciate why that person may have behaved like that, or perhaps acknowledge that if you had been in that situation you might have had a similar response. This revised point of view, which enables you to move away from your initial assumptions or judgments, should link into your formal knowledge of your subject area. You may be prompted to think about the skill of empathy or the importance of effective communications skills (see Chapter 2), or indeed a consideration of questions about professional behaviour and values.

Within this section you should note the attempt to begin to theorise your experience, linking your analysis to an attempt to make better sense of the experience by drawing on the knowledge sources of your subject area and so demonstrating learning.

'Now what?' is the level of working with this revised or enhanced understanding. As an action plan, your reflections prompt you to read more about the importance of empathy and person-centred approaches to working therapeutically (see the work of Rogers (1967), for example). Alternatively if your analysis of the event centred around your anxiety and exploring in more detail these feelings, your 'now what?' may reveal the need for more support in helping you deal more effectively with situations that provoke your anxiety by identifying coping strategies that enable you to deal more successfully with such situations.

Moon's (1999) work covers five stages:

1. Noticing: this is the descriptive stage of your writing – as Moon points out, learners will only learn something if they notice it (Moon, 1999, p141).

2. Making sense: this represents the beginning stage of analysis – here you are trying to put some structure or coherency to your initial thoughts and feelings about the event in question. You are trying to make sense of the situation/experience, by asking: What does this mean? Why did I think that? Why did I behave like that? Why do I feel like this?

3. Making meaning: this stage goes a step further than the initial analysis of making sense as you begin to think about how your initial analysis of events links into what you already know – it is the stage of theorising as you draw upon the range of knowledge sources you know to develop your understanding. Moon (1999) suggests that, at this stage, the learner is demonstrating deep learning as ideas are being linked together and there is evidence that a more holistic view of the subject area is developing (p143).

4. Working with meaning: at this stage, Moon suggests that a number of cognitive processes are utilised, such as critical analysis, thoughtful reasoning and making a judgment. The ability to give appropriate explanations seems to be a good indicator of functioning at this stage (p145). You are now actively engaging and using the knowledge sources of your subject area to inform and enhance your work or practice – there is confidence in what you know, based upon a critical understanding of the subject and you are able to demonstrate and use this knowledge with ease in your academic work or in a practice setting.

5. Transformative learning: at this stage, reflection on your learning becomes even more sophisticated and learners are able to demonstrate *that they are capable of evaluating their frames of references, the nature of their own and others' knowledge and the process of knowing itself . . . A learner at this stage will be self-motivating and self-motivated* (p146). At this stage, the reflective learner may express their understanding in comments such as *my outlook has changed and I am critical of the whole of our approach. Let me explain how* (Moon, 1999, p146).

For both this and the previous stage of reflective learning, engaging in the process of critical analysis and deep attempts at meaning-making requires a deliberate and conscientious effort at processing and making sense of the learning or event. It involves reading and rereading texts, revision of learning and discussions in tutorials or with practice mentors to generate ideas and question the topic – hence the emphasis on being self-motivated and taking responsibility for your own learning.

The final model of reflection is based on the work of Gibbs (1988) and covers six stages of the reflective process.

1. description of events;
2. feelings and thoughts: here the emphasis is on self-awareness;
3. evaluation: at this stage, you are making a judgment about what happened; what was good or bad about the event; what went well or not so well;
4. analysis: here you are asking deeper questions about your evaluation – it is the stage of examination and interrogation from different perspectives and drawing on your formal knowledge sources;
5. conclusion: having explored the situation in more detail and from different perspectives, you now have more information to make a more informed judgment about what went on. This is the stage of revised insight or understanding and provides the opportunity to learn from your experience;
6. action plan: your revised understanding or new insight is used to help you think about your future practice or learning; how can you use this new understanding to improve your performance in the future?

Whilst Borton's (1970) work might seem the simplest because there are only three stages, for all the models there is likely to be movement between all the stages rather than viewing each stage as discrete and not blurring into one another. In addition, remember that these are only models: they are meant to be useful for helping you structure your thinking for reflective purposes, so try not to see the models as prescriptive. You may find an aspect of Moon's (1999) model useful whilst Gibbs' (1988), with its separate focus on feelings and thoughts, is a useful prompt for remembering that exploration of emotions and feelings is an important part of the reflective process.

> ### ACTIVITY 6.4
> Use Borton's model to write a reflective account about a significant learning experience, using his three prompts of: What? So what? Now what?

Comment

Look at the list below, which identifies key elements of reflective writing and compare the list to your own account from Activity 6.4 and see if it incorporates these points.

Drawing on the work of Walker (2008), the following list identifies what should be included in reflective writing:

- builds upon a description of an event/experience;
- is exploratory;
- uses critical thinking skills to analyse the event in depth and examine it from different perspectives;
- uses formal theory, research, knowledge and values to enhance understanding;
- has an emotional content;
- can be challenging and uncomfortable;
- promotes change as part of the learning process.

(adapted from Walker, 2008, p98)

CHAPTER SUMMARY

- Critical reflection is an aid to developing a deep approach to learning.
- It is defined as a structured approach to thinking about a significant event or experience that involves interrogating and analysing it from different viewpoints.
- Reflection is an aid to learning and self-development and should aim to improve your understanding of yourself, your practice experiences and your classroom learning.
- In aiming to make sense and improve your understanding, you should also draw upon established knowledge sources to aid your development.
- The reflective practitioner also recognises the importance of learning from practice placements and is able to demonstrate learning from these experiences.
- Three different models of reflection have been suggested that can be used to help structure and organise your thinking for a reflective account of your learning experiences.

FURTHER READING

Rolfe, G, Jasper, M and Freshwater, D (2010) *Critical Reflection in Practice* (2nd edition). Hampshire: Palgrave.

This provides a systematic coverage of reflection. It includes a useful chapter on developing reflective writing and is written to appeal to the health and social welfare student and practitioner.

Thompson, S and Thompson, N (2008) *The Critically Reflective Practitioner.* Hampshire: Palgrave.

This book, written to appeal to a variety of health and social care practitioners and students at different levels of study, is accessible and informative.

Conclusion

In this book, we have highlighted the range of key skills that you need to develop in your studies to achieve a successful outcome at university or in practice. At undergraduate level you are expected, by the end of your studies, to show that you have a general knowledge of your subject area. Your lecturer cannot teach you everything you need to know for that purpose. Whilst good universities provide a variety of teaching and learning strategies to support and engage students in their learning, you are still expected to take increasing responsibility for your own learning through private study and critical analysis of your understanding. Whilst your tutor and the university student support services will provide support and guidance, at the end of the day, you have to produce the work to meet the assessed requirements for your course.

As the first chapter shows, learning to learn at higher education level is so important. A deep approach to learning is expected – an approach where you show evidence of being able to make sense and understand the new learning material over the long term and how this applies to a variety of contexts. Consequently, developing effective communication skills is vital within academic work and on your practice placements. Chapters 2–4 cover the range of communication skills that are necessary to develop in order to achieve successful outcomes both in your studies and with people you work with when you go out on placement.

However, as the title of the book suggests, study skills need to be practised and developed so that you become confident in their use. Engagement with the learning activities and reflective exercises in each chapter can help cultivate these skills and put them into practice. Several case studies are included to show the link between your reading and practice.

Practice learning opportunities provide a vital link between university learning and the 'real world' and these are necessary for you to demonstrate that you can put into practice what you have been learning about. This is covered in Chapter 5, as is the link between the knowledge, skills and values that you are expected to demonstrate whilst on placement.

The final chapter on reflection has brought you back to the importance of learning and being able to demonstrate your understanding of what you have learnt. Reflection is a cognitive process of trying to make sense of a learning experience or incident in order to improve your understanding through critical analysis of the experience. You reflect in order to enhance your understanding and improve your learning and practice. Critical reflection is evidence of a deep approach to learning and, again, through having engaged with the learning activities you should feel able to develop your reflective abilities and show evidence of your learning.

Undertaking a degree is a challenge and makes demands on your time. It requires self-discipline, and perhaps surprisingly, self-centredness, since at degree level you are investing time, energy and money in this venture and presumably you want a return – not least, to be successful. By working your way through this book and undertaking the learning activities, you should be able to use your new understanding to inform your studies and be confident that you are on your way to a successful conclusion. Your commitment to the process of learning means you can feel proud of your achievements. We wish you good luck on your learning journey and your development towards being a successful qualified practitioner in the helping professions.

Glossary

Accreditation of prior learning (APL) APL allows credit for previous learning and experience, usually in the form of an exemption from part of a course. This is normally assessed by learners providing evidence that they have met the learning outcomes of the module from which they want to be exempt.

Active learning see **learning**.

Active listening The word 'active' is used to emphasise that effective listening is a *mental activity that requires effort and concentration* (Williams, 1997, p47).

Admissions tutor The person responsible for selecting successful applications to a particular course.

Alternative Languages and Augmentative Communication Systems The recognition that not all people speak and not all body language is commonly used or understood throughout the world. Languages can be non-verbal, such as sign language, or alternative systems such as Makaton and image communication. Written communication can take the form of characters that are not the recognisable letters of the Roman alphabet, for example Braille and the Moon alphabet.

Assessment The process of checking and marking your coursework. Depending on your course, assessments may include examinations, essays, project work, reports or a combination of any of these (see **formative assessment** and **summative assessment**).

Assessment board Also known as an exam board, an assessment board is a meeting of the academic staff and the external examiners to agree the marks for each student (see **award board** and **module board**).

Award The outcome or result of your course, including a degree, certificate or diploma.

Award board A meeting of the academic staff and the external examiners to agree the award for each student or to agree that a student can progress to the next part of the programme. Award boards and assessment boards can occur concurrently.

BA Bachelor of Arts (see **Bachelor's degree** and **BSc**).

Bachelor's degree Undergraduate degree qualification awarded by the university. It can take the form of an ordinary degree (BA or BSc) or an Honours degree (BA(Hons) or BSc(Hons)).

BSc Bachelor of Science (see **BA** and **Bachelor's degree**).

Bursary A financial grant given to eligible students by some **PSRBs** that doesn't need to be repaid.

Campus The university buildings and facilities in a particular location.

Careers service Provides expert information and advice on career prospects, including help in developing a CV and finding work.

Certificates Qualifications usually leading to the Certificate of Higher Education. A certificate is issued following the completion of a one-year course.

Communication skills These include verbal, written, presentational, non-verbal, individual and group skills (see **non-verbal communication** and **verbal communication**).

Competencies Skills and knowledge that are essential to perform the functions of the profession successfully.

Core unit/module Course unit or module that is compulsory or required and must be completed successfully in order to gain an award.

Coursework A piece of work you need to complete as part of your course.

CRB (Criminal Records Bureau) Enhanced checks are undertaken for all professional programmes where students are working with vulnerable adults or children to ensure their suitability for practice placements and protection of the public.

Critical reflection see **reflection**.

Degree Typically three years' full-time or four to six years' part-time study, leading to the university award of Bachelor or Master.

Degree classification The grading scheme for undergraduate degrees. Honours degrees can be first-class, upper (2:1) and lower (2:2) second-class, or third-class honours.

Deep learning see **learning**.

Department Many university faculties or schools are divided into departments, for example, Department for Social Studies. Students belong to the department that provides the course on which they are enrolled.

DipHE/Diploma of Higher Education An award given for successfully completing two years' full-time study at the university.

Dissertation A major written piece of work or research project undertaken in the final year of an undergraduate Honours degree course.

ECDL European Computer Driving Licence – a scheme for assessing ICT competence.

Enrolment The process where students become registered students of the university. This must be done at the beginning of every year.

Essay A written piece of work on a particular topic.

Ethics In contrast to values, ethics is more prescriptive and deals with what can be considered 'right and correct'. Ethics represents guidelines or principles about the way professionals ought to behave, and many helping professionals have codes of ethics or codes of conduct to which members are expected to adhere and to which they can be held to account (see **values**).

Exams officer The member of the academic staff responsible for collating all student results and presenting them to an exam board.

Extenuating circumstances A procedure whereby students can ask for particular circumstances that may have affected their studies to be taken into account, particularly in relation to assessment (see **mitigating circumstances**).

Faculty A collection of schools and departments in a university, for example, Faculty of Health and Social Studies.

Feedback The range of feedback comments that you receive from your tutor/module leader and your practice teacher/mentor intended to aid your learning and facilitate improvement. This can refer to feedback in class following a learning activity; feedback on performance in your placement; feedback in an individual tutorial; as well as formative and summative feedback on your work (see **assessment**).

Formative assessment Designed to provide learners with feedback on progress and inform development. A draft of your work that does not contribute to the overall assessment outcome (see **assessment** and **summative assessment**).

Foundation degree Involves study at university or college and work-based learning. A foundation degree is completed at level 5 of the academic framework, that is, at the equivalent level to the second year of a Bachelor's degree.

Fresher Student in the first few weeks of study.

Freshers' week A week of events and activities for new students before their studies; organised by the Students' Union.

Graduand Student who has completed his or her studies and who is awaiting graduation.

Graduate Someone who has successfully completed a degree programme and who has completed graduation at the university.

Graduation ceremony Takes place at the end of your studies; degrees are awarded. You will be able to invite a small number of guests.

Halls Halls of residence or accommodation for students.

Higher education Post compulsory education. Higher education courses are usually studied at universities, university colleges and higher education institutions. They can also be studied at specialist colleges, for example, art and music, and some further education colleges.

Honours (Hons) degree A full British undergraduate degree that usually requires completion of a final-year dissertation or research project and the achievement of 360 credits.

ICT Information and communication technology.

Information literacy Your ability to recognise why information is needed, what information is needed, how to access this information and how to evaluate it (see Table 3.1 highlighting the SCONUL model).

Interrupt The process whereby students can have a break in their studies, usually due to unforeseen circumstances.

IT help desk An important resource when dealing with your ICT needs; located in your university/college.

Learning At higher education level, deep approaches to learning are encouraged. Learning is about understanding the subject material and promotes long-term retention of the information that can be applied in the 'real world'. It represents an active approach to managing your learning coupled with a motivation to understand the subject. In contrast, surface or superficial learning concentrates more on the 'here and now'. This approach to learning tends to promote rote learning or the memorisation of key facts or information, but fails to link the new material to the wider picture.

Learning outcomes What a student is expected to know and demonstrate at the end of a particular module. Learning outcomes should then be assessed by the summative assessment associated with the module of study.

Lecture A presentation on a particular subject or topic given by a member of the academic staff to a large number of students. Generally, students listen and take notes.

Lecturers (or tutors) Lecturers and tutors are members of the university academic staff and are responsible for teaching and learning and helping students with their studying.

Level Level 4 refers to the first year of a university course, level 5 to the second year and level 6 to the third year. Part-time students will take longer to complete each level than full-time students. Postgraduate courses begin at level 7.

Lexicon The vocabulary necessary to communicate in any context. The wider your lexicon, the better the potential outcomes for your studies and practice.

MASTER A mnemonic for motivate, acquire, search, trigger, exhibit, reflect. A useful strategy to help you develop your thinking skills.

Master's degree A postgraduate academic degree awarded by a university upon completion of at least one year of prescribed study beyond the Bachelor's degree.

Mature student A student who is 21 years of age or over.

Mitigating circumstances A procedure where students can ask for particular circumstances that may have affected their studies to be taken into account, particularly in relation to assessment (see **extenuating circumstances**).

Module A unit of study that is worth a number of credits, for example, 10, 15, 20 or 30 credits. Typically students undertake 120 credits in a year so the number of modules you study depends on the credit value, for example, six modules of 20 credits each equals 120 credits.

Module board A meeting of the academic staff and the external examiners to agree the marks for each student.

Module leader The lecturer responsible for the delivery, assessment and review of a module of study.

Module specification/guide Details of the module or unit of study which is provided by the module leader outlining what will be covered during the course of study; the learning outcomes associated with the module; how students will be assessed in their learning; and further reading/reading lists.

National occupational standards (NOS) A set of requirements for which you are required to demonstrate competence in relation to your practice placements over the duration of your studies.

Non-verbal communication Anything other than words or utterances that are used to convey a message or meaning. This involves body language, including posture, gestures and expressions and even how you dress (see **verbal communication**).

NUS National Union of Students. On enrolment you will be issued with an identity card that acts as your student union card.

Off-site practice assessor/tutor/mentor Someone who supports you on work placement but who is not based in the same agency. This person works with another member of staff within your placement to offer support and guidance and to assess your competence against the national occupational standards (see **practice teacher**).

Option unit/module Course unit that is chosen by the student from a number of alternatives.

Ordinary degree A Bachelor's degree awarded for the achievement of approximately 300 credits.

Placement A period of relevant work experience designed to give students an opportunity to meet the requirements for the programme and the national occupational standards.

Plagiarism Citing someone else's work in your written work and failing to acknowledge it through proper referencing or acknowledgment. Academically, this is cheating and even committed inadvertently is still an offence. In the most serious of cases, this can result in a student's studies being terminated.

Postgraduate Study that is beyond first degree level or Bachelor's level, and leads to a higher qualification such as a Master's degree or Doctorate.

Practice teacher/assessor/mentor A qualified practitioner within your placement to offer support and guidance and to assess your competence against the national occupational standards.

Programme Set of units that lead to an award. Sometimes referred to as a course.

Programme leader Member of academic staff responsible for managing the programme or course you are studying.

PSRB Public Statutory Regulatory Body, a quasi governmental agency with responsibilities for regulating professionals and their practice, including registration of professionals.

Reflection A structured approach to thinking that looks back on an experience or event that has occurred. It is a cognitive activity that involves the mental process of selection, attention and analysis in order to develop or deepen our understanding of something and therefore enhance our capacity to know or do something (action) differently in the future.

Reflective practitioner Being able to demonstrate your learning about professional practice during your placements in health, social welfare or educational settings. To be reflective in your placement settings is, therefore, about how you demonstrate your learning from this experience – it transforms an experience into knowledge because your experience has been of benefit to you and as a result you can show evidence of learning from it.

Registration You may be required to register with the PSRB. Registration is also the term used by the university at enrolment. You will need to register for your course at the beginning of each academic year.

Seminar Small-group teaching, led by a tutor/module leader where students are expected to come prepared to participate and share their learning and understanding, following private study and reading which has been set by the tutor.

Service user or **user of service** Those members of the public with whom you will work when on placement or in employment.

SQ3R An approach to reading and study that involves the process of survey, question, read, recall and review.

Summative assessment Assessment designed to be used to determine grades or marks (see **assessment** and **formative assessment**).

Supervision Provides a vital role in supporting and managing your practice while you are on placement. It should be an educative and supportive process, supporting you in your learning and understanding of your professional development.

Surface learning see **learning**.

Teaching and learning strategies The range of teaching and learning activities that are used in your programme to help engage you in your learning and support your understanding of the subject matter, for instance, case studies, group work, lectures and seminars.

Term A period of study in the academic year, for example, from October to December.

Tuition fees Money paid each year by students to enrol or attend a course.

Tutor or lecturer A member of staff who is responsible for teaching and learning and helping students with their studying.

Tutorial A study session during which an individual, or small group, meets with a tutor in order to discuss work, progress or general course issues.

Undergraduate A student who is studying for a Bachelor's degree. Someone who has already been awarded a degree from a university is known as a graduate.

Undergraduate degree A course of study or programme of research leading to a Bachelor's degree.

Union A shortened name for the Students' Union.

Values Representative of general preferences and which shape our beliefs and attitudes. They tend to represent what can be described as good and desirable or worthwhile. They influence behaviour and have an affective quality as well; that is, they have an impact on our emotions. Professional bodies also tend to have a set of professional values to which members are expected to practise (see **ethics**).

Verbal communication This includes words and utterances. We convey meaning through pitch, tone of voice, volume and speed of speech, or noises (see **non-verbal communication**).

References

Anderson, L and Krathwohl, D (eds) (2001) *A Taxonomy for Learning, Teaching, and Assessing: A revision of Bloom's Taxonomy of Educational Objectives*. New York: Longman.

Bandura, A (1977) *Social Learning Theory*. London: Prentice-Hall.

Banks, S and Gallagher, A (2008) *Ethics in Professional Life: Virtues for health and social care*. Basingstoke: Palgrave Macmillan.

Beauchamp, T L and Childress, J F (1994) *Principles of Biomedical Ethics*. New York: Oxford University Press.

Bloom, B S, Engelhart, M D, Furst, E J, Hill, W H and Krathwohl, D R (1956) *Taxonomy of Educational Objectives: The classification of educational goals. Handbook I: Cognitive domain*. New York: Longmans, Green.

Bolton, G (2005) *Reflective Practice: Writing and professional development*. London: Sage.

Borton, T (1970) *Reach, Teach and Touch*. London: McGraw Hill.

Brown, K and Rutter, L (2006) *Critical Thinking for Social Work*. Exeter: Learning Matters.

Bruce, C, Edwards, S and Lupton, M (2006) Six Frames for Information literacy Education: a conceptual framework for interpreting the relationships between theory and practice. The Higher Education Academy Information and Computer Sciences ejournal: *Italics*, 5: issue 1.

Burnard, P (1997) *Effective Communication Skills for Health Professionals* (2nd edition). Cheltenham: Nelson Thornes.

Burns, T and Sinfield, S (2003) *Essential Study Skills* (2nd edition). London: Sage.

Buzan, T and Buzan, B (2006) *The Mind Map Book – Full illustrated edition*. London: BBC Books.

Cottrell, S (2011) *Critical Thinking Skills* (2nd edition). Basingstoke: Palgrave.

Damasio, A (1999) *The Feeling of What Happens: Body, emotion and the making of consciousness*. London: Heinemann.

Datta, S and MacDonald-Ross, M (2002) Reading skills and reading habits: a study of new Open University undergraduate reservees. *Open Learning: The Journal of Open and Distance Learning*, 17 (1): 69–88.

Edwards, S and Bruce, C (2006) Panning for gold: understanding students' information searching experiences, in Bruce, C, Mohay, G, Smith, G, Stoodley, I and Tweedale, R (eds) *Transforming IT Education: Promoting a culture of excellence*. Santa Rosa, California: Informing Science.

Fry, H, Ketteridge, S and Marshall, S (2001) Understanding student learning, in Fry, H, Ketteridge, S and Marshall, S (eds) *A Handbook for Teaching and Learning in Higher Education.* London: Kogan Page.

General Social Care Council (2010) *Codes of Practice for Social Care Workers*. London: GSCC.

Gibbs, G (1988) *Learning by Doing: A guide to teaching and learning methods*. Oxford: Oxford Further Education Unit.

Goleman, D (1998) *Working with Emotional Intelligence.* London: Bloomsbury.

Griffiths, S (1999) Teaching and learning in small groups, in Fry, H, Ketteridge, S and Marshall, S (eds) *A Handbook for Teaching and Learning in Higher Education*. London: Kogan Page.

Hanley, P (2009) Communication skills in social work, in Adams, R, Dominelli, L and Payne, M (eds) *Social Work, Themes, Issues and Critical Debates* (3rd edition). Basingstoke: Palgrave.

Healey, J and Spencer, M (2008) *Surviving Your Placement in Health and Social Care: A student handbook.* Berkshire: OU Press.

HM Government (2005) *Common Core of Skills and Knowledge for the Children's Workforce.* Nottingham: DCSF.

Hounsell, D (2007) *Not Written for Us?* Keynote speaker, 7th Annual Learning and Teaching Conference, University of Teesside.

Howarth, J (2010) See the practitioner, see the child: the framework for the assessment of children in need and their families ten years on. *British Journal of Social Work*, 41: 1070–1087.

Howe, D (2009) *A Brief Introduction to Social Work Theory*. Basingstoke: Palgrave.

Knott, C and Scragg, T (2007) *Reflective Practice in Social Work.* Exeter: Learning Matters.

Koprowska, J (2005) *Communication and Interpersonal Skills in Social Work*. Exeter: Learning Matters.

Lishman, J (1994) *Communication in Social Work*. Basingstoke: Macmillan Press.

Lupton, M (2004) *The Learning Connection: Information literacy and the student experience.* Adelaide: Auslib Press.

Marton, F and Saljo, R (1997) Approaches to learning, in Marton, F, Hounsell, D and Entwistle, N (eds) *The Experience of Learning*. Edinburgh: Scottish Academic Press.

McCarthy, P and Hatcher, C (2002) *Presentation Skills: The essential guide for students.* London: Sage.

Mayer, J D and Salovey, S (1997). What is emotional intelligence?, in Salovey, P and Sluyter, D (eds) *Emotional Development and Emotional Intelligence: Educational implications*. New York: Basic Books.

Mezirow, J (1991) *Transformative Dimensions of Adult Learning.* San Francisco: Jossey Bass.

Millar, M and Corby, B (2006) The framework for the assessment of children in need and their families – a basis for a 'therapeutic' encounter? *British Journal of Social Work,* 36: 887–899.

Miller, S and Sambell, K (eds) (2003) *Contemporary Issues in Childhood: Approaches to teaching and learning*. Newcastle: Northumbria University Press.

Moon, J (1999) *Reflection in Learning and Professional Development.* Abingdon, Oxon: RoutledgeFalmer.

National Committee of Inquiry into Higher Education (The Dearing Report) (1998) *Higher Education in the Learning Society*. Available online: www.leeds.ac.uk/educol/ncihe/.

National Youth Agency (NYA) (2008) *Professional and National Occupational Standards for Youth Work*. Leicester: NYA.

Nursing and Midwifery Council (2008) *The Code: Standards of conduct, performance and ethics for nurses and midwives*. London: NMC.

Oko, J (2011) *Understanding and Using Theory in Social Work* (2nd edition). Exeter: Learning Matters.

Quality Assurance Agency for Higher Education (2008) *The Framework for Higher Education Qualification in England, Wales and Northern Ireland.* Mansfield: QAA.

Ramsden, P (2003) *Learning to Teach in Higher Education* (2nd edition). London: Routledge.

Rogers, C (1967) *On Becoming a Person: A therapist's view of psychotherapy.* London: Constable.

Rose, C and Nicholl, M (1998) *Accelerated Learning for the 21st Century.* New York: Bantam Doubleday Dell.

Rothman, J C (1998) *From the Front Lines: Student cases in social work ethics.* Boston: Allyn & Bacon.

SCONUL Advisory Committee on Information Literacy (1999) *Briefing Paper: Information skills in higher education.* London: Society of College, National and University Libraries. Available online: www.sconul.ac.uk/groups/information_literacy/papers/Seven_pillars2.pdf

Sheppard, M (2007) Assessment: from reflexivity to process knowledge, in Lishman, J (ed) *Handbook for Practice Learning in Social Work and Social Care.* London: Jessica Kingsley.

Thompson, N (2006) *Anti-discriminatory Practice* (4th edition). Basingstoke: Palgrave.

Thompson, N (2009) *People Skills* (3rd edition). Basingstoke: Palgrave.

Walker, H (2008) *Studying for Your Social Work Degree.* Exeter: Learning Matters.

Williams, D (1997) *Communications Skills in Practice: A practical guide for health professionals.* London: Jessica Kingsley.

Yorke, M (2004) Employability in higher education: what it is – what it is not, in *Learning and Employability. Series One.* York: Enhancing Student Employability Co-Ordination Team/ Higher Education Academy.

Useful websites

www.hpc-uk.org Health Professions Council: regulates social work in England and many of the professions allied to medicine in the UK.

The following bodies regulate social work in the devolved countries:

www.ccwales.org.uk Care Council for Wales.

www.niscc.info Northern Ireland Social Care Council.

www.sssc.uk.com Scottish Social Services Council.

www.collegeofsocialwork.org College of Social Work.

www.nmc-uk.org Nursing and Midwifery Council: the nursing and midwifery regulator for England, Wales, Scotland, Northern Ireland and the islands.

www.nya.org.uk National Youth Agency: works in partnership with government, private and voluntary sector organisations to support and improve services for young people.

www.rcn.org.uk Royal College of Nursing: represents nurses and nursing, promotes excellence in practice and shapes health policies.

Index

absolutistic view of knowledge and learning 8
accountability 77–8, 79
accreditation of prior learning (APL) 99
active listening 19, 27, 29–30, 99
admissions tutor 99
aim/purpose of a presentation 58, 61–2
Alternative Languages and Augmentative
    Communication Systems 31, 99
analysis 41, 43
AND 41
anxiety 13
   dealing with in presentations 65–7
application 11, 43
argument, developing an 36–7
assessment 15, 99
assessment board 99
assessment outcomes 19–20, 33
audience (of presentation) 58, 62–3
award 99
award board 99

Bachelor's degrees 99–100
background emotions 23
Banks, S. 75
biases 41
body language 19, 29, 31, 63
   see also non-verbal communication
Bolton, G. 84, 85
books, referencing 52
Boolean operators 41
Borton, T. 93, 95

breathing exercises 66
Bruce, C. 35
Burnard, P. 23–4
bursaries 100

campus 100
Care Standards Act 2000 72
careers service 100
case studies 16
categories of learning 8
certificates 100
chapters in a book, referencing 52
clarity 26
codes of practice/codes of ethics 70–1, 72, 73
cognitive and intellectual skills (assessment
    outcome) 20
College of Social Work 70, 72
common morality approach 75
communication skills 3, 18–32, 34, 59–60, 97,
    100
   active listening 19, 27, 29–30, 99
   alternative communication approaches 31
   ethics and employability 77, 79
   importance of 19–20
   non-verbal communication 19, 22–5, 63,
    103
   rules of communication 20–1
   verbal communication 19, 25–9, 104
   see also presentation skills
competence 70
competencies 100

concept cards 28–9
concern, genuine 77, 79
concrete experience 89
confidentiality 81
consultation, ongoing 80
context, and communication 21, 25
core modules/units 14, 100
Cottrell, S. 86, 89
course of study/programme 103
    beginning 15–17
    choosing 12–14
coursework 100
CRB (Criminal Records Bureau) checks 100
creating skills 43
critical approach to learning 8
critical reflection 85–7
    see also reflection

data collection methodology 42
databases 38, 40
Dearing Report 19
decision-making 70–1
    ethical theories and 75–6
deep learning 2, 9–11, 76, 84, 97, 102
    promoting 12–14
deep reading 48–9
degree classification 100
degrees 100
    Bachelor's 99–100
    foundation 1, 14, 101
    honours (Hons) 101
    Master's 102
    ordinary 103
    undergraduate 104
Department of Children, Schools and Families
    59
departments 100
dictionaries 28–9, 49
difficult work situations 90
DipHE (Diploma of Higher Education) 100
dissertation 100
drafting 54
'Dublin descriptors' 59
dyslexia 54–5
dyspraxia 54–5

ECDL (European Computer Driving Licence)
    100

editing 54
Edwards, S. 35
emotional intelligence 34, 35, 36–7
emotions 22–3
empathy 77, 79
employability 70, 71
    development as an employable practitioner
        77–8, 79
empowerment 77–8, 79
engaging a listener 63
enrolment 13, 100
entry qualifications 14
essays 100
    writing 47–55
ethics 70–1, 74–8, 101
    development as an ethical practitioner
        77–8, 79
    ethical dilemmas 76
    ethical theories and decision-making 75–6
evaluation skills 43
evidence, seeking 37
exams officer 101
experience 89–90
    bridge between theory and 89–90
    concrete 89
extenuating circumstances 101
eye contact 31

faculty 101
family commitments 14
feedback 16–17, 54, 101
first year of the course 14
fitness to practise 70
footnote (Vancouver) referencing system 51
formal presentations 57
formative assessment 101
formative feedback 16, 54
foundation degrees 1, 14, 101
foundation year 14
freshers 101
freshers' week 101
Fry, H. 7

Gallagher, A. 75
General Social Care Council 59
Gibbs, G. 94–5
graduands 101
graduates 101

graduation ceremony 101
grammar 53
group discussions 11, 16
group presentations 67–8
group work 14, 16, 87–8

halls of residence 101
Hanley, P. 30
Harvard referencing system 51–2
Hatcher, C. 64
Health Professions Council 59, 71
higher education 101
Higher National Diplomas (HNDs) 1, 14
higher-order thinking skills 42–4
honesty 77, 79
honours (Hons) degrees 101
Howarth, J. 75

index card system 50
induction programme 13
informal presentations 57
information and communication technology
    (ICT) 3, 33, 34–41, 47, 101
    finding information and literature 38–41
information literacy 34–7, 101
information sources 38–40
interaction, communication and 21
internet searches 35, 38–41
interrupt (interruption process) 102
involvement of the service user 77, 79
IT help desk 102

journals 49
    referencing 52
justice 75

Kant, I. 75
key transferable skills 20
keywords 40–1
knowledge and understanding (assessment
    outcome) 20

learning 2, 5–17, 84, 102
    deep learning 2, 9–11, 12–14, 76, 84, 97,
        102
    definition 5–7, 8
    preparing to study 9–11
    relationship to teaching 9, 12

student approaches to 7–8
    surface learning 9–11, 12, 48, 76, 84, 102
    transformative 36, 94
learning agreement 80
learning difficulties 54–5
learning environments, safe 30
learning outcomes 15, 102
learning and teaching strategies 15–17, 104
lecture notes 11
lecturers 102, 104
    see also tutors
lectures 102
levels of study 102
lexicon 26–8, 47, 102
links, making 11
Lishman, J. 22
listening, active 19, 27, 29–30, 99
lower-order thinking skills 42–4
Lupton, M. 36–7

Marton, F. 9
MASTER mnemonic 44–5, 102
Master's degrees 102
mature students 102
Mayer and Salovey four-branch model of
    emotional intelligence 36–7
McCarthy, P. 64
meaning-making 6, 7, 36, 87, 94
memorisation 9
mentor, practice 78–80, 103
mind maps 45–6, 53
mitigating circumstances 102
models of reflection 92–5
module board 102
module guides/specifications 15, 102–3
module leaders 14, 15, 102
modules 102
Moon, J. 36–7, 87, 93–4, 95
morals 70–1, 74
    see also ethics
motivation 1–2, 6–7, 12–13

National Committee of Inquiry into Higher
    Education Report (Dearing Report) 19
national occupational standards (NOS) 70, 72,
    103
National Youth Agency 71–2
nerves 65–7

Nicholl, M. 44–5
non-discriminatory behaviour 81
non-verbal communication 19, 22–5, 63, 103
   recognising non-verbal behaviours 24–5
   self-awareness of 23–4, 25
NOT 41
notes
   lecture notes 11
   reading notes 49–50
noticing 37, 93
Nursing and Midwifery Council 59, 71
NUS (National Union of Students) 103, 104

objectives of a presentation 61–2
off-site practice assessor/tutor/mentor 78–80, 103
Office for Standards in Education, Children's Services and Skills 72
open days 13
option unit/module 103
OR 41
ordinary degrees 103
outcomes
   assessment outcomes 19–20, 33
   learning outcomes 15, 102

pace 63
paralinguistics 29
partnership working 77–8, 79
peer group learning 87–8
peer-reviewed journals 49
personal life 14
personal tutors 14
photographs 88
pitch 63
placements see practice learning
plagiarism 50, 103
planning
   presentations 60–1
   writing 53–4
poster presentations 67
postgraduate study 103
practical and professional skills (assessment outcome) 20
practice, for a presentation 63
practice learning 3, 69–82, 89–90, 97, 103
   employability 70, 71, 77–8, 79
   ethical and moral decision-making 70–1

preparing for placement 78–82
professional bodies 71–4
thinking about ethical behaviour 74–8
practice teacher/assessor/mentor 78–80, 103
preparation
   for placement 78–82
   for a presentation 60–1
presentations 3, 56–68
   audience 58, 62–3
   dealing with nerves and anxiety 65–7
   engaging the listener 63
   formal and informal 57
   group presentations 67–8
   necessity for 59–60
   planning and preparation 60–1
   poster presentations 67
   process 58
   purpose of 61–2
   structure 64–5
professional bodies 71–4
Professional and National Occupational Standards for Youth Work 59
professionalism 60, 70, 79, 81
programme see course of study/programme
programme leader 103
proofreading 53
Public Statutory Regulatory Bodies (PSRBs) 70, 71–2, 74, 75, 103
punctuation 53
purpose/aim of a presentation 58, 61–2

Quality Assurance Agency for Higher Education (QAA) 59

Ramsden, P. 8
reading 3, 27, 34, 47–50
   deep approach 48–9
   difficulties with 54–5
   notes 49–50
   referencing and plagiarism 50–2
   with a purpose 48–9
reciprocal processing 58
referencing 50–2
reflection 2, 3, 83–95, 97–8, 103
   critical 85–7
   definition 83–5
   importance 87–8
   in supervision 90–1

information literacy 35, 36–7
  models of 92–5
  role of supervision 90
  writing reflectively 91–2, 95
reflective practitioner 88–90, 103–4
reflective recordings/diary 81
reflexivity 85–7
register of qualified practitioners 72
registration 104
relativistic conception of learning and
  knowledge 8
relaxation techniques 65
remembering skills 43
research 62–3
responsibility 81
role-plays 16
Rose, C. 44–5
rote learning 9
Rothman, J.C. 75
rules of communication 20–1

safe learning environments 30
Saljo, R. 8, 9
Salovey, S. 36–7
sample size and representativeness 41
searches for information 35, 38–41
self-awareness about non-verbal
  communication skills 23–4, 25
self-efficacy 2
seminars 16, 104
sense-making 37, 94
service users 104
  involvement 77, 79
  partnership working with 77–8, 79
sign languages 31
simplicity 26
slides, presentation 64–5
social responsibility, learning as a 36
social self 23
Society of College, National and University
  Libraries (SCONUL) skills for
  information literacy 35, 36–7
spell checkers 53
SQ3R approach 49–50, 104
staged models of reflection 93–5
structure
  presentations 64–5
  verbal communication 26

student population diversity 7
student support services 13, 14
studying 9
subject gateways 38
subject-specific dictionaries 28, 49
summative assessment 104
summative feedback 16, 54
supervision 90–1, 104
  ongoing 80
  reflection in 90–1
support for students 13, 14
surface learning 9–11, 12, 48, 76, 84, 102
SWOT analysis 78, 80
symbolic communication 22
syntax 53

Teaching Agency 71, 72
teaching–learning relationship 9, 12
teaching and learning strategies 15–17, 104
terms 104
thesauri 28
thinking skills 33, 41–6
  lower-order and higher-order 42–4
  strategies for thinking 44–6
Thompson, N. 29–30
time management 14
tone 63
trade unions 73, 74
transferable skills, key 20
transformative learning 36, 94
transition to higher education 2, 5–17
  beginning the course 15–17
  choosing a course 12–14
trust 77, 79
tuition fees 104
tutorials 104
tutors 34, 38, 81, 102, 104
  admissions tutor 99
  off-site practice assessor/tutor/mentor
    78–80, 103
  personal tutors 14

undergraduate degrees 104
undergraduates 104
understanding 9, 11, 43, 58, 87
union (National Union of Students) 103, 104
universal emotions 22–3
utility 75

values 70–1, 74, 104
Vancouver referencing system 51
verbal communication 19, 25–9, 104
virtue ethics 75
vocabulary 26–8, 47, 102
vocational qualifications 14

Walker, H. 95
websites, referencing 52

workplace-based learning 89–90
    see also practice learning
writing 3, 34, 50–5
    difficulties with 54–5
    process 53–4
    referencing and plagiarism 50–2
    reflective writing 91–2, 95

zone of fantasy 23